Praise for
Skinny **Bitch**

"A funny, foul-mouthed ode to adopting a vegan diet."
—Dwight Garner, *New York Times Book Review*

"The authors are brazen . . . They're not trying to win
popularity contests . . . they just want healthy people."
—Associated Press News Syndicate

"Ready to jump-start [the year] with an electric prod to the system? . . .
They tell it like it is, and without delicacy."
—*Chicago Sun Times*

"There's more solid advice in *Skinny Bitch* than in most diet and health books."
—*Bitch Magazine*

"By no means for the faint hearted . . . this is as hard hitting as it comes!"
—*Hot Stars* (UK)

"This diet book doesn't sugar-coat what you have to do to lose weight."
—*Grazia*

"It made me laugh . . ." —*Marie Claire UK*

"Sensible advice . . ." —*Health & Fitness UK*

" . . . an absolutely hilarious read . . . refreshingly in-your-face funny. . . .
What are you waiting for, you moron? Go buy this book!"
—*Florida Today*

"What makes this diet easy to swallow is the book's tough-love attitude—
part best-friend counsel, part drill-sergeant abuse and a dash of
sailor mouth, wrapped in a pretty chick-lit package."
—iVillage, Diet & Fitness

Skinny
Bitch
In the Kitch

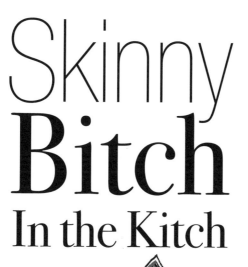

Kick-ass recipes for
hungry girls who want
to stop cooking crap
(and start looking hot!)

by Rory Freedman and Kim Barnouin

RUNNING PRESS
PHILADELPHIA · LONDON

9 8 7 6 5 4 3 2 1
Digit on the right indicates the number of this printing

Library of Congress Control Number: 2007933176

ISBN: 978-0-7624-3542-5

Book design by Amanda Richmond
Edited by Jennifer Kasius
Typography: Bodoni and Helvetica Neue

This book may be ordered by mail from the publisher.
Please include $2.50 for postage and handling.
But try your bookstore first!

Running Press Book Publishers
2300 Chestnut Street
Philadelphia, PA 19103-4371

Visit us on the web!
www.runningpress.com

To the truth-speakers and seekers who paved the way for us,
For the health food pioneers who blazed a trail for us to follow,
For our fellow foodies who love to eat as much as we do,
And for all the newly hatched Skinny Bitches who asked for this book.

Namastè.

CONTENTS

ACKNOWLEDGMENTS

Jill Hough, we cannot imagine what this book would be without your passion, dedication, and culinary brilliance. Thank you! Talia Cohen, Jennifer Kasius, Amanda Richmond, Seta Bedrossian Zink, Craig Herman, and Victoria Gilder: For your ceaseless support and enthusiasm and for everything you do (including the things you do that we'll never even know about), we express our sincerest gratitude. Really. We are so thankful for each of you. For creating the perfect *Skinny Bitch*, we will forever be indebted to you, Margarete Gockel. Chloe Jo Berman, Talia Berman, Karen Coyne, Meri Freedman, Bruce Friedrich, Jessica Jonas, Dave and Linda Middlesworth, Jack Norris, Steve Perron, Gretchen Ryan, Lauren and Tracy Silverman, and everyone at VTM: Your commitment and generosity leave us in awe. And to everyone at Laura Dail Literary Agency, Perseus Books, and Running Press: We humbly thank each of you for being part of the collective that makes this all possible. We don't take any of you for granted.

For our friends and families, who make the whole journey a joy—we couldn't ask for more.

INTRODUCTION

What's better than eating? (If you say "sex," you're either a liar or a pervert.) The answer is: Nothing! There's nothing better than eating! We're total pigs and eating is, without a doubt, our favorite thing to do. We love eating so much, it makes us mad. We have, like, a violent passion for food. When we go out to eat, if something we order is really good, we talk about killing the chef. Or our pets. Or ourselves. Good food makes us want to die . . . you know, like that expression, ". . . to die for." But ironically, we also care about our health.

It was these two things—our obsessive passion for food and our concern for health—that led us to write *Skinny Bitch*. If you haven't read *Skinny Bitch* yet, get your head out of your ass and go buy a copy. It will change your life. Seriously. Don't be fooled by the title; it's not some dumb, fluffy, weight-loss book. It's a comprehensive guide on how to eat well *and* enjoy food. But it's also a well-researched exposé documenting the shady business surrounding what we eat.

Much of what we learned while researching *Skinny Bitch* blew our minds. So we've made it our personal mission to share this information. We wanted to reprint *Skinny Bitch* in its entirety right here in the introduction, but our whore publisher wouldn't let us. So we're gonna give you the Cliff Notes . . .

Meat:

Hmm . . . dead, rotting, decomposing flesh of carcasses. Doesn't sound like something you'd want to eat, huh? Not to mention the pesticides, hormones, steroids, and antibiotics. Oops! We almost forgot mad cow disease, bird flu, salmonella, E. coli, trichinosis, and mercury. Well, no wonder Americans are suffering from obesity; cancer; liver, kidney, lung, and reproductive disorders; birth defects; miscarriages; and nervous system disorders.

You can call it steak, tuna, bacon, or chicken. No matter how you slice it, it's a piece of decaying, decomposing carcass. We know you like the taste, but there are other foods out there that mimic the flavor and texture of meat but don't come with the same side effects. Smarten up, bitches.

Dairy:

Got osteoporosis? Researchers at Harvard, Yale, Penn State, and the National Institutes of Health have studied the effects of dairy intake on bones. Not one of these studies found dairy to be a deterrent to osteoporosis. On the contrary, a study funded by the National Dairy Council itself revealed that the high protein content of milk actually leaches calcium from the body. These findings are consistent with many others that blame milk not only for osteoporosis, but also acne, anemia, anxiety, ADD, allergies, asthma, obesity, heart disease, diabetes, autism, and multiple cancers.

Just like human milk is for baby humans, cows' milk is for baby cows. We're the only species on the planet that drinks the milk of another species. We're also the only species on the planet that drinks milk as adults. It's not only gross, it's creepy. We've been totally duped by the dairy industry and their hundreds of millions of advertising dollars. And now we're totally addicted to their disease-causing products.

There's no need for any of them. It's the new millennium. There are so many awesome alternatives to dairy products. Get with the program, bitches.

Carbs:

There is so much bullshit around carbs now; we've got to set the record straight. There are two types of carbs—simple and complex. Complex carbs are not only good for you, but they're a vital part of your diet. They consist of fruits, vegetables, whole grains, and legumes, and they should be eaten all day, every day. Simple carbs suck and should be avoided: white bread, white flour, white pasta, white rice, and white sugar. Most cookies, cakes, snacks, and processed foods are simple carbs.

So what's a pig to do? Have her cake and eat it—just make the cake with good ingredients. Duh!

Whenever we do interviews promoting *Skinny Bitch,* we're always asked the same questions: "What do you do when you get cravings for cookies? Or does that never happen to Skinny Bitches?" Um, we're Skinny Bitches, not aliens! Of course we get cravings for cookies. And when we do, we eat 'em!

Unfortunately, most people have no idea that they can truly enjoy food without getting fat, sick, or sad. So it's our pleasure (oink, oink) to educate and feed the masses. We hope you'll love these recipes as much as we do. If you don't, go have sex, you pervert.

Bitchclaimer

There's nothing more annoying than recipes with a million obscure ingredients. So we tried to make all our recipes as "normal" as possible. However, there are a few products we insist on using, despite their potential to peeve you. You may not have whole wheat flour lying around in your cupboard, but too bad. White flour is crap for your body and should only be used when absolutely necessary. Whenever we can, we use products that are as pure and healthy as possible. And we want the same for you. We want you to replace your old, shitty ingredients and start eating better.

Now granted, there's nothing wrong with olive oil. In fact, we love it. But did you know that when you heat most oils at high temperatures, you change their molecular structures, causing free-radicals? And that free-radicals have been linked to heart disease and cancer? Well, we knew that (we're really smart), so a lot of our recipes call for coconut oil instead. Yeah, you may have to go to a health food store to buy it, but isn't a trip to the health food store better than a trip to the Emergency Room?

So if you come across a few ingredients that irritate you: Don't hate. Appreciate. We love you and we want you to enjoy food *and* be healthy. We have a glossary in the back to explain some of the funky stuff. So quit your bitching, restock your cabinets, and get cookin'.

(Don't worry, though—there are some naughty, crappy ingredients in here, too.)

Bitchin'
BREAKFASTS

*Coffee sucks for your body and is no way to start
your day. (If that's news to you, go read* Skinny Bitch,
*pages 15–16.) The real breakfast of champions is
fresh fruit. But for weekend brunches and those days when
fruit ain't gonna cut it, enjoy these bitchin' breakfasts.*

French Scramble

Homemade Granola Parfait

THE Breakfast Sandwich

Potato Scramble

Pecan-crusted French Toast

Basic Pancakes

Basic Fruit and Nut Muffins

Smoothies

Bitchin' Breakfast Burrito

Denver Bitchlette for Two

French Scramble

Serves 3 or 4

14 to 16 ounces firm or extra firm tofu,
   crumbled (use your hands or a fork)

4 ounces vegan Jack, cheddar,
   or American cheese, shredded

3 scallions, sliced

2 cloves garlic, minced

2 tablespoons nutritional
   yeast flakes

1 tablespoon tamari or soy sauce

½ teaspoon turmeric

½ teaspoon fine sea salt

½ teaspoon pepper

½ tablespoon refined
   coconut oil

1 cup sliced mushrooms
   (any kind, or a combination)

2 cups fresh spinach leaves

In a large bowl, combine the tofu, cheese, scallions, garlic, yeast flakes, tamari or soy sauce, turmeric, salt, and pepper. Set aside.

In a large nonstick skillet over medium heat, melt the coconut oil. Add the mushrooms and cook, stirring occasionally, until tender, about 1½ minutes. Stir in the spinach, a handful at a time if necessary, and cook until wilted, about 1 minute. Stir in the tofu mixture and cook, stirring occasionally, for 3 to 4 minutes, or until any liquid has evaporated and the mixture is hot. Serve immediately.

Homemade Granola Parfait

Makes 1

1 cup berries (if using strawberries, hull and quarter them)

1 (6-ounce) container vanilla or fruit-flavored soy yogurt

⅔ cup homemade granola

HOMEMADE GRANOLA

Makes about 6 cups

2 cups rolled oats

1¼ cups (4 ounces) sliced almonds

¾ cup unsweetened shredded coconut

¼ teaspoon fine sea salt

¼ cup maple syrup

2 tablespoons rice syrup

2 tablespoons safflower oil, plus more for greasing baking sheet

1 cup dried fruit (raisins, golden raisins, cranberries, chopped apricots — use just one or any combination you want)

Preheat oven to 300°F.

Arrange the oats on a large rimmed baking sheet and bake, stirring occasionally, until lightly toasted, about 15 minutes.

Meanwhile, in a large bowl, combine the almonds, coconut, and salt. In a small bowl, whisk together the maple syrup, rice syrup, and oil.

Stir the toasted oats into the almond mixture. Add the syrup mixture, stirring to thoroughly combine.

Grease the baking sheet. Spread the granola evenly on the sheet and bake, stirring occasionally, until golden brown, 20 to 25 minutes (the mixture will still look and feel wet). Stir in the dried fruit, then cool completely in the pan on a wire rack. (It'll be torturous waiting for it to cool. But do your best. This bitch is hot.) Store in an airtight container.

THE Breakfast Sandwich

Makes 4

1 (7- or 8-ounce) package
   baked or fried tofu (2 squares)

2 tablespoons refined coconut oil

4 slices vegan Canadian bacon
   or ham

4 slices vegan Jack, cheddar,
   or American cheese

4 whole wheat English muffins,
   split and toasted

4 slices tomato (optional)

2 tablespoons soy butter

Fine sea salt

Pepper

Ketchup (optional)

Halve both of the tofu squares crosswise, making 4 patties. In a large skillet over medium heat, melt the coconut oil. Add the tofu and bacon or ham and cook 2 minutes. Turn both and add a small amount of soy butter to the tofu before topping the tofu with the cheese. Cover and cook another 2 minutes. On each of the 4 muffin bottoms, arrange 1 slice of bacon or ham, 1 piece of tofu with cheese, and 1 slice of tomato, if using. Sprinkle generously with salt and pepper, add ketchup if desired, and add the muffin tops. Serve immediately. Then die happy.

Potato Scramble

Serves 4 to 6

8 ounces vegan Jack, cheddar, or mozzarella cheese, shredded

7 to 8 ounces firm or extra firm tofu, cut into ½-inch dice

2 tomatoes, cut into ½-inch dice

1 teaspoon fine sea salt

½ teaspoon pepper

½ teaspoon paprika

1 tablespoon refined coconut oil

8 ounces vegan breakfast sausage, crumbled or cut into small bite-sized pieces

½ onion, cut into ½-inch dice

2 russet potatoes (about 24 ounces), cut into ½-inch dice

2 cloves garlic, thinly sliced

In a large bowl, combine the cheese, tofu, tomatoes, salt, pepper, and paprika; set aside.

In a large nonstick skillet over medium heat, melt ½ tablespoon of the coconut oil. Add the sausage and cook according to package directions. Transfer the sausage to the bowl with the cheese mixture. Add the remaining ½ tablespoon of coconut oil to the skillet and melt over medium heat. Add the onion and cook, stirring occasionally, for 1 minute. Add the potatoes and cook, stirring occasionally, until the potato is tender, 15 to 20 minutes. Stir in the garlic and cook for 1 minute. Stir in the cheese mixture and cook, stirring occasionally, for 2 to 3 minutes, or until the mixture is hot.

Pecan-crusted French Toast

Makes 6 to 8 slices

1½ cups soy or rice milk

3 tablespoons corn starch

1 teaspoon cinnamon

6 tablespoons chickpea flour
   or brown rice flour

1 cup finely chopped pecans

2 tablespoons refined coconut oil,
   or more as needed for cooking

6 to 8 slices vegan whole wheat
   or whole wheat raisin bread

Maple syrup, for serving

In a medium bowl, whisk together the soy or rice milk, corn starch, and cinnamon. Whisk in the chickpea or brown rice flour. Transfer the mixture to a shallow bowl. Place the pecans in another shallow bowl.

In a large skillet over medium heat, melt the coconut oil. One slice at a time, dip the bread in the milk mixture, turning to soak both sides. Dip one side in the pecans, pressing to coat. (Yeah, it's a little challenging to make 'em stick in there. Quit whining. You're about to have French toast!) Arrange the bread in the skillet (you might have to do more than one batch), pecan side down. Cook 2 to 3 minutes, until the pecans are well browned. Carefully turn the bread and continue cooking until the second side is browned, 2 to 3 minutes. Serve immediately with maple syrup.

Basic Pancakes

Makes about eight

4- to 5-inch pancakes

1¼ cups whole wheat pastry flour

1½ teaspoons baking powder

½ teaspoon fine sea salt

1½ cups rice milk

2 tablespoons refined coconut oil,
   melted, or safflower oil

1 tablespoon maple syrup,
   plus more for serving

1 teaspoon pure vanilla extract

In a large bowl, whisk together the flour, baking powder, and salt. In a medium bowl, whisk together the rice milk, oil, maple syrup, and vanilla. Whisk the milk mixture into the flour mixture, stirring just until combined (a few lumps are okay).

Preheat a nonstick griddle or large nonstick skillet over medium heat for at least 2 minutes. About ¼ cup at a time, pour the batter onto the grill or skillet. Cook until bubbles appear, the edges are set, and the pancakes are nicely browned on the bottom (about 2 to 3 minutes). Turn and cook until the other side is nicely browned, 1 to 2 minutes. If necessary, keep the finished pancakes in a warm oven while you finish the batter. Serve hot with maple syrup.

BLUEBERRY PANCAKES

Stir 1 cup of blueberries into the batter.

BANANA WALNUT PANCAKES

Stir 1 large banana, thinly sliced, and ½ cup chopped walnuts into the batter.

CHOCOLATE PANCAKES

Reduce the whole-wheat pastry flour to 1 cup plus 2 tablespoons. Add ¼ cup unsweetened cocoa powder. Increase the syrup to 2 tablespoons.

Basic Fruit and Nut Muffins

Makes 12 standard-sized muffins

¼ cup refined coconut oil, melted, or safflower oil, plus more for greasing muffin tins

2 cups whole wheat pastry flour

½ cup Sucanat or other dry sweetener

1 tablespoon Ener-G egg replacer

2 teaspoons baking powder

¼ teaspoon fine sea salt

1¼ cups soy milk

1 teaspoon vanilla

1 cup fresh or dried fruit, diced or chunked, if necessary

½ cup chopped nuts (optional)

Preheat oven to 375°F. Grease a standard-sized muffin tin or use muffin liners.

In a large bowl, combine the pastry flour, Sucanat, baking powder, salt and egg replacer. In a medium bowl, whisk together the soy milk, oil, and vanilla. Add the milk mixture to the flour mixture, stirring until barely combined. Stir in the fruit and nuts, if using. Transfer the batter to the prepared muffin tin, dividing it evenly. Bake for 15 to 20 minutes, or until a toothpick inserted into the center of the muffins comes out clean.

CRANBERRY ORANGE MUFFINS

Add the zest of ½ orange. Use dried cranberries for the fruit and omit the nuts.

TROPICAL MACADAMIA NUT MUFFINS

Add the zest of ½ orange, combine banana and shredded coconut for the fruit, and use macadamias for the nuts.

APPLE CINNAMON MUFFINS

Use apples for the fruit, omit the nuts, and add 1 teaspoon ground cinnamon, ¼ teaspoon ground nutmeg, and ⅛ teaspoon ground cloves to the dry ingredients.

ZUCCHINI RAISIN MUFFINS

Combine shredded zucchini and raisins for the fruit, omit the nuts, and add 1 teaspoon ground cinnamon and ½ teaspoon ground ginger to the dry ingredients.

Basic Fruit Smoothie

Makes about 2 cups

2 cups chunked, frozen fruit
(see note)

1 cup soy milk or juice OR ½ cup
soy milk and ½ cup juice

In a blender, combine the fruit and soy milk and/or juice. Puree until smooth.

> If using fresh fruit, just add ½ cup ice cubes.

STRAWBERRY BANANA SMOOTHIE

Use a banana and strawberries for the fruit, and all soy milk for the liquid.

VERY BERRY SMOOTHIE

Use mixed berries for the fruit, and half soy milk, half apple juice for the liquid. (Or you can use all soy milk.)

JUST PEACHY SMOOTHIE

Use peaches for the fruit, and half soy milk, half apple juice for the liquid.

TROPICAL ORANGE GINGER SMOOTHIE

Use banana for the fruit, and orange juice for the liquid; add 1 tablespoon minced fresh ginger.

Bitchin' Breakfast Burrito

Makes 4

14 to 16 ounces firm or extra firm tofu,
  crumbled (use your hands or a fork)

2 cloves garlic, minced

2 tablespoons nutritional yeast flakes

1 tablespoon tamari or soy sauce

½ teaspoon turmeric

1 teaspoon fine sea salt

½ teaspoon pepper

1 tablespoon refined coconut oil

8 ounces vegan breakfast sausage,
  crumbled

1 russet potato (about 12 ounces),
  cut into ½-inch dice

1 (15-ounce) can black or pinto
  beans, drained

1 (4-ounce) can diced green chiles,
  drained

4 (9- to 10-inch) whole wheat tortillas,
  heated

4 ounces vegan cheddar or Jack
  cheese, shredded

1½ to 2 cups salsa

In a large bowl, combine the tofu, garlic, yeast flakes, tamari or soy sauce, turmeric, salt, and pepper; set aside.

In a large nonstick skillet over medium heat, melt ½ tablespoon of the coconut oil. Add the sausage and cook according to package directions. Transfer the sausage to the bowl with the tofu mixture. Add the remaining ½ tablespoon of coconut oil to the skillet and melt over medium heat. Add the potato and cook, stirring occasionally, until tender, 12 to 15 minutes. Add the beans and chiles, stirring until heated through, about 1 minute. Stir in the tofu mixture and cook, stirring occasionally, for 3 to 4 minutes, or until any liquid has evaporated and the mixture is hot.

To serve, lay a tortilla on a work surface and top with ¼ of the tofu mixture, arranging it in a column down the middle of the tortilla, 2 inches from either edge. Top with ¼ of the cheese and ¼ cup of the salsa. Fold one side of the tortilla up and over the fillings, fold in the edges, and continue rolling the tortilla to the other side, making a tight bundle. Transfer the burrito to a plate, seam down. Repeat with remaining tortillas. Pass the remaining salsa at the table. Olé, bitches!

Denver Bitchlette for Two

Serves 2

9 to 10 ounces firm or extra firm tofu, crumbled (use your hands or a fork)

3 ounces vegan Jack, cheddar, or American cheese, shredded

2 cloves garlic, minced

4 teaspoons nutritional yeast flakes

2 teaspoons tamari or soy sauce

2 teaspoons Ener-G egg replacer

½ teaspoon turmeric

½ teaspoon fine sea salt

½ teaspoon pepper

1 tablespoon refined coconut oil

½ green bell pepper, cut into ¼-inch dice

½ red bell pepper, cut into ¼-inch dice

¼ onion, cut into ¼-inch dice

1 slice or about 1 ounce vegan Canadian bacon or ham, cut into ¼-inch dice

Paprika for garnish (optional)

In a large bowl, combine the tofu, cheese, garlic, yeast flakes, tamari or soy sauce, egg replacer, turmeric, salt, and pepper. Set aside.

In a large nonstick skillet over medium heat, melt ½ tablespoon of the coconut oil. Add the green bell pepper, red bell pepper, and onion and cook, stirring occasionally, until tender, about 3 minutes. Transfer the vegetables to a plate or bowl.

Return the skillet to medium heat and melt the remaining ½ tablespoon of coconut oil. Add the tofu mixture and cook, stirring occasionally, for 2 minutes. Then spread it evenly in the pan and cook, without stirring, until nicely browned on the bottom, 2 to 3 minutes.

Arrange the vegetable mixture and bacon or ham on top of one side of the omelet. Remove from the heat and gently slide the omelet about halfway onto a serving plate. Carefully turn the pan over to fold the omelet in half on the plate.

Don't get all cranky if you screw up folding the Bitch-lette. It's definitely a talent that takes time to develop.

If you want, sprinkle the omelet with paprika before serving.

PMS
PISSY MOOD
SNACKS

*If a group of scientists conducted a study
saying PMS wasn't "real," we'd kill them all.
Then we'd stuff our faces like sows.
This is what we'd eat.*

Quesadillas

"Ham" and Cheese Puff Pockets

Onion Rings

Oven-Baked Garlic Fries

Quick Tortilla Pizzas

Quesadillas with Beans, Soy Cheese, Guacamole, and Salsa

Serves 2 as an entree

or 4 as an appetizer

½ tablespoon refined coconut oil (optional)

2 (9- or 10-inch) whole wheat flour tortillas

5 ounces vegan Jack or cheddar cheese (or a combination), shredded

⅓ cup drained black or pinto beans

½ cup prepared salsa

¼ cup guacamole, homemade or store bought (recipe follows)

Spread the coconut oil, if using, on one side of each tortilla, dividing it evenly. Lay the tortillas, oiled side down if applicable, on a work surface. Arrange the cheese on top, dividing it evenly, covering only half of the tortilla and leaving a 1-inch border at the edge. Arrange the beans and 2 tablespoons of the salsa on top of the cheese, dividing them evenly. Fold the tortillas in half.

In a large nonstick skillet over medium heat, cook the quesadillas, covered, until golden brown, about 4 minutes. Flip the quesadillas and cook, uncovered, until the second side is golden brown and the cheese has melted, about 2 minutes. Cut the quesadillas in wedges and transfer to serving plates or a platter. Top with guacamole and a spoonful of the remaining salsa. Pass any leftover salsa at the table.

GUACAMOLE

Makes about 1 cup

1 medium avocado

1 clove garlic, minced or pressed

Juice of ½ lime (about 1 tablespoon)

½ teaspoon fine sea salt

In a small bowl, use a potato masher or fork to combine the avocado, garlic, lime, and salt, stirring to make a coarse purée. Use immediately.

"Ham" and Cheese Puff Pockets

Makes 4

Whole wheat pastry flour,
    for dusting work surface

2 (9-inch) vegan whole wheat pie
    crusts, room temperature

4 ounces vegan cheddar cheese,
    shredded

4 ounces vegan sliced ham

Preheat oven to 400°F. Line a rimmed baking sheet with parchment.

On a work surface lightly dusted with whole wheat pastry flour, combine both pie crusts and roll them into a 12 x 12-inch rectangle. Cut the pastry in quarters to make four 6-inch squares. Top the squares with about half of the cheese, dividing evenly, covering only half of the pastry and leaving a ¾-inch border at the edge. Fold or cut the ham to cover the cheese, dividing evenly. Place the remaining cheese on top of the ham, dividing evenly.

Fold the pastry in half, pressing the edges together to seal in the filling. Crimp the edges with a fork. Prick the pocket a few times to create air vents. Transfer the pockets to the prepared baking sheet and bake for 20 minutes or until nicely browned.

Onion Rings

Makes about 20 rings

Refined coconut oil,
   for greasing baking sheet

1 onion (preferably a sweet
   type), cut crosswise into
   ⅓-inch-thick slices

½ cup seasoned whole
   wheat bread crumbs

½ cup cornmeal

1 teaspoon fine sea salt,
   plus more for sprinkling

¾ cup rice flour

¾ cup soy or rice milk

Ketchup, or other dipping
   sauce (optional)

Preheat oven to 450°F. Grease a large rimmed baking sheet; set aside.

Separate the onion slices into rings and pick out 20 or so of the largest (reserve the rest for another use). In a shallow bowl, combine the bread crumbs, cornmeal, and salt. Place the rice flour in a second bowl and the soy milk in a third. One at a time, dip the onion rings in the soy milk, the rice flour, the soy milk again, and then the bread crumb mixture, pressing to thoroughly coat. Arrange the coated rings on the prepared baking sheet and bake for 25 to 30 minutes, or until nicely browned. Sprinkle with salt and serve with ketchup, if desired.

Oven-baked Garlic Fries

Serves 3 or 4

2 russet potatoes, scrubbed, peeled (if desired), and cut into ¼-inch sticks

4½ tablespoons refined coconut oil, melted, or safflower oil

4 cloves garlic, minced

Fine sea salt

1 teaspoon chopped fresh parsley (optional)

> * Don't be cheap with the baking sheets, even though you might be able to squeeze them onto just one. More room around the fries helps them crisp.

Preheat oven to 450°F.

In a large bowl, combine the potatoes with 3 tablespoons of the oil, tossing to coat evenly. Arrange the potatoes on two* large rimmed baking sheets in a single layer and bake for 15 minutes. One pan at a time, remove the fries from the oven and flip them over with a spatula. Rearrange the fries in a single layer and return them to the oven for 15 to 20 minutes, until crisp outside and cooked through.

Meanwhile, in a small saucepan over low heat, combine the remaining 1½ tablespoons of oil and the garlic. Cook, stirring occasionally, until the garlic is fragrant and starting to brown, about 3 minutes.

Transfer the fries to serving plates or a platter. Sprinkle generously with salt and drizzle with the garlic mixture. Sprinkle with parsley, if desired.

Quick Tortilla Pizzas

Makes 4

4 (9- to 10-inch) whole wheat tortillas

1 cup Roasted Red Pepper Sauce
  (recipe below)

4 to 6 ounces vegan mozzarella,
  shredded

½ small red onion, thinly sliced

⅓ cup halved and pitted
  Kalamata olives

2 cups loosely packed arugula,
  (optional)

Preheat oven to 475°F.

Arrange tortillas on two rimmed baking sheets. *

Top the tortillas with the Roasted Red Pepper Sauce, cheese, onion, and olives, dividing evenly. Bake for 8 to 10 minutes, until the cheese is bubbly and the edges are brown.

Cut the pizzas into quarters, top with the arugula, if using, and serve.

ROASTED RED PEPPER SAUCE

Makes 1 cup

1 cup drained jarred roasted
  red peppers

6 large basil leaves

¼ teaspoon fine sea salt

⅛ teaspoon pepper

In the bowl of a food processor, combine the roasted red peppers, basil, tomato paste, salt, and pepper; pulse to form a coarse paste.

> * For crispy pizza, bake the tortillas for 3 minutes, flip 'em and bake 'em for 3 minutes more. Then, add the toppings and bake for 8 to 10 minutes.

Grown-up
APPETIZERS

If we were having a dinner party
and pretending to be classy,
we'd make stuff like this.

Crabby Cakes with Remoulade Sauce

Garlicky White Bean Spread on Crostini

Herbed "Egg" Salad Scoops

Mock Chopped Liver

Spicy Mixed Nuts

Stuffed Mushrooms

Spicy Sushi Rolls
with Avocado and Cucumber

Crabby Cakes with Remoulade Sauce

Serves 8 as an appetizer

(or 4 as an entrée)

About 2 tablespoons refined
   coconut oil

1 cup diced carrots

½ cup diced celery

4 shallots, minced

2 cups finely shredded parsnip

1 cup whole wheat panko
   (Japanese-style bread crumbs)
   or whole wheat bread crumbs

¼ cup chickpea flour
   or brown rice flour

2 tablespoons Ener-G egg replacer

4 teaspoons kelp powder

1½ teaspoons fine sea salt

¼ teaspoon pepper

½ cup vegan mayonnaise

About 1 cup Remoulade Sauce
   (recipe follows)

In a large nonstick skillet, heat 1 tablespoon of the coconut oil. Add the carrots and celery and cook over medium heat, stirring occasionally, for 2 minutes. Add the shallots and cook, stirring occasionally, for 1 minute, or until all the vegetables are tender. Remove from heat and allow to cool.

In a mixing bowl, combine the parsnip, panko, flour, egg replacer, kelp powder, salt, and pepper. Stir in the carrot and celery mixture and mayonnaise. Shape the mixture into 8 cakes, about 3 inches across and ¾ inch thick.

Wipe out the skillet and return it to medium heat. Add the remaining tablespoon of coconut oil. When the oil is hot, add the cakes and cook until golden brown, 2 to 3 minutes per side. (Don't crowd the skillet; you might have to do more than one batch.) Serve immediately drizzled with Remoulade Sauce.

REMOULADE SAUCE

Makes about 1 cup

1 cup vegan mayonnaise

2 tablespoons lemon juice

2 tablespoons finely chopped chives

1 tablespoon Dijon mustard

1 tablespoon prepared horseradish

1 tablespoon tomato paste

1 tablespoon sweet paprika

½ teaspoon fine sea salt

¼ teaspoon white pepper

In a medium bowl, whisk together the mayonnaise, lemon juice, chives, mustard, horseradish, tomato paste, paprika, salt, and pepper. Set aside in the refrigerator until ready to serve.

Serve the cakes on a simple mixed green salad dressed with a lemony vinaigrette.

Garlicky White Bean Spread on Crostini

Makes about 40 bite-sized appetizers

1 (15-ounce) can cannellini beans, drained

2 to 4 cloves garlic

3 tablespoons lemon juice

1 tablespoon extra virgin olive oil

¼ teaspoon fine sea salt, or more to taste

⅛ teaspoon pepper

2 teaspoons chopped fresh Italian parsley, basil, or a combination

Additional chopped fresh Italian parsley or basil, or diced roasted red peppers, for garnish (optional)

About 40 crostini, homemade (recipe follows) or store bought

In the bowl of a food processor, combine the beans, 2 cloves of garlic, lemon juice, olive oil, salt, and pepper. Puree, stopping to scrape the bowl as needed. Taste and add more garlic or salt as desired. Stir in the 2 teaspoons of chopped parsley and/or basil.

Top each crostini with about 2 teaspoons of the bean spread. Top the spread with a sprinkle of chopped herbs or a couple of pieces of diced peppers, if desired. Arrange crostini on a platter and serve.

If you don't feel like laboring over 40 appetizers, serve the bean spread in a bowl and arrange the crostini alongside.

CROSTINI

Makes 40 crostini

10 slices whole wheat bread
   or 1 baguette

Refined coconut oil,
   melted (optional)

Preheat oven to 350°F.

If using bread, trim off the crusts and cut each slice into quarters. If using a baguette, cut it diagonally into about 20 slices, then cut each slice in half. Brush the bread with the coconut oil, if desired.

Arrange the bread in a single layer on 1 or 2 large rimmed baking sheets. Bake for 8 to 15 minutes, depending on the bread, until dry and slightly browned. Cool before using.

Herbed "Egg" Salad Scoops

Makes about 40 appetizers

Makes about 40 appetizers

5 large heads endive

14 to 16 ounces extra firm tofu,
   drained and pressed (to squeeze
   out excess water)

¼ small diced white onion
   (about ¼ cup)

¼ cup vegan mayonnaise

1 tablespoon Dijon mustard

1½ tablespoons lemon juice

1 teaspoon fine sea salt

¼ teaspoon white pepper

¼ teaspoon curry powder

1 tablespoon chopped fresh chives

1 tablespoon chopped fresh parsley

2 teaspoons chopped fresh tarragon

Separate the endive leaves, setting aside about 40 (reserve the rest for another use).

In a large bowl, crumble the tofu. Stir in the onion, mayonnaise, mustard, lemon juice, salt, pepper, and curry powder. Add about 2 teaspoons of the chives, about 2 teaspoons of the parsley, and about 1 teaspoon of the tarragon.

About 1 tablespoon at a time, place a scoop of salad onto the tip of each endive leaf. Arrange the leaves on a platter, sprinkle with the remaining herbs, and serve.

Mock Chopped Liver

Makes about 2 cups

2 tablespoons refined coconut oil

1 onion, cut into rough ½-inch dice

1 pound cremini (brown)
   mushrooms, thickly sliced

3 cloves garlic, roughly chopped

1 cup raw cashews, toasted

2 tablespoons nut oil, such as
   walnut or hazelnut, or extra
   virgin olive oil

1 tablespoon Bragg's Liquid
   Aminos, or more to taste (or two
   teaspoons tamari or soy sauce)

1 teaspoon fine sea salt,
   or more to taste

¼ teaspoon pepper, or more to taste

Heat the coconut oil in a large skillet over medium-high. Add the onions and cook, stirring occasionally, until they just begin to brown, about 3 minutes. Add the mushrooms and cook, stirring occasionally, until the mushrooms are limp and the released liquid has almost entirely evaporated, 8 to 10 minutes. Stir in the garlic and cook for 1 minute. Set aside to cool.

In a food processor, pulse the cashews until finely chopped. Add the mushroom mixture, nut oil, Bragg's Liquid Aminos, salt, and pepper and process until smooth. Add more Bragg's Liquid Aminos, salt, and/or pepper to taste.

> It's good enough to eat with a spoon, but serve it on crackers or something.
> Be a lady.

Spicy Mixed Nuts

Makes about 3 cups

1½ teaspoons Ener-G egg replacer

2 tablespoons warm water

1 pound roasted, salted mixed nuts

⅓ cup evaporated cane sugar

2 teaspoons kosher
   or other coarse salt

1½ teaspoons cayenne powder

Do not eat entire batch in
one sitting. Seriously.

Preheat oven to 250°F.

In a medium bowl, whisk the egg replacer and water until foamy. Add the nuts and toss to coat. Transfer the nuts to a strainer and let drain for at least 2 minutes.

Meanwhile, wipe out the bowl and combine the sugar, salt, and cayenne. Add the nuts, tossing to coat. Spread the nuts in a single layer on a large rimmed baking sheet. Bake for 40 minutes. Stir with a spatula and spread the nuts out again. Reduce the oven to 200°F and bake another 30 minutes, or until dry. The nuts will crisp as they cool to room temperature. Thoroughly cooled, they can be stored for up to one week in an airtight container.

Stuffed Mushrooms

Makes 20 mushrooms

2 tablespoons refined coconut oil,
   plus more for greasing baking sheet

20 large (2 to 2 ½ inches across)
   white mushrooms

1 red bell pepper, finely diced

1 shallot, finely diced

½ teaspoon dried oregano

6 tablespoons whole wheat
   seasoned or Italian bread crumbs

6 tablespoons vegan
   Parmesan cheese

¼ cup chopped fresh Italian parsley

1 teaspoon fine sea salt

½ teaspoon pepper

Preheat oven to 400 ° F. Grease a large, rimmed baking sheet.

Carefully pull the stems from the mushroom caps; set stems aside. Arrange the caps, stem sides down, on the prepared baking sheet and bake until they leak liquid, about 10 minutes. Remove from the oven and set aside.

While the caps are baking, finely chop the stems. Heat the oil in a large skillet over medium-high. Add the stems and cook, stirring occasionally, until golden brown, 2 to 3 minutes. Add the bell pepper, shallot, and oregano and cook, stirring occasionally, until the bell pepper is tender, about 3 minutes. Transfer the mixture to a medium bowl to cool slightly, then stir in the bread crumbs, cheese, parsley, salt, and pepper.

Turn the mushroom caps over and spoon in the filling, pressing gently and slightly mounding it. Bake until the mushrooms are tender and the stuffing is browned, about 20 minutes. Then eat every last one before anyone else can try them.

Spicy Sushi Rolls with Avocado and Cucumber

> If you're short on patience or easily frustrated, you're better off going to your local Japanese restaurant. There is a Zen art to making sushi rolls, and if you're cursing and screaming and carrying on, your sushi will sucky.

Makes 4 rolls

¼ cup vegan mayonnaise

½ to 1 tablespoon sriracha (or other chili sauce; see note), or more to taste

4 sheets nori (see note)

About 3 cups prepared Brown Sushi Rice (recipe follows)

1 avocado, peeled, pitted, and sliced

½ small cucumber, peeled, halved lengthwise, seeded, and sliced lengthwise

½ small carrot, julienned

Soy sauce for serving

Wasabi paste for serving (see note)

Pickled ginger for serving (see note)

Special equipment: bamboo sushi mat (see note)

In a small bowl, combine the mayonnaise with ½ tablespoon of sriracha. Taste and add more sriracha if you like.

Place a bamboo sushi mat on a clean work surface, with the sticks in the mat parallel to you. Place a sheet of nori on the mat, shiny side down, shorter edge toward you. Have a shallow bowl of water nearby. Dampen your hands in the water, shaking off the excess moisture. Use your fingers to press about ⅔ cup of Sushi Rice onto the nori, covering ⅔ of the sheet closest to you (if the rice sticks to your hands as you work, redampen them in the water). Drizzle about 1 table-spoon of the mayonnaise mixture on top of the rice in a line parallel to you, about

1 inch in from closest edge. Top the mayonnaise with ¼ of the avocado, ¼ of the cucumber, and ¼ of the carrots.

Take a deep breath and smile. Holding the fillings firmly in place with the fingertips of both hands, use both thumbs to lift the edge of the mat closest to you up and over, enclosing the fillings. Squeeze gently to make a compact roll. Raise the end of the mat slightly to avoid rolling it in with the nori, and continue rolling, squeezing occasionally, until the sushi is completely rolled in to a tight cylinder. If necessary, dampen the end of the nori to help it seal, then allow the roll to sit for a minute or two. Slice the roll into 8 pieces with a sharp, lightly moistened knife. Repeat with the remaining ingredients, making 4 rolls total. Serve the sushi on a platter with soy sauce, wasabi, and pickled ginger.

SRIRACHA (an Asian chili sauce), NORI (seaweed sheets), WASABI paste, and PICKLED GINGER can be found in the Asian section of most major supermarkets.

Look for a BAMBOO SUSHI MAT there, too, or in the utensils section, or at cookware stores. Before you start, cover the sushi mat with plastic wrap to make it easy to clean.

Brown Sushi Rice

Makes about 3 cups

1 cup short-grain brown rice
  (see note)

2 cups water

3 tablespoons seasoned
  rice vinegar (see note)

Sushi rice is traditionally made with white rice, but we're health rebels!

Seasoned rice vinegar can be found in the Asian section of most major supermarkets.

In a 2-quart saucepan over high heat, combine the rice and water. Bring to a boil, reduce the heat to a simmer, cover, and cook until the water is absorbed and the rice is tender, about 45 minutes. Remove from the heat and let the rice stand, covered, at least 10 minutes.

Turn the cooked rice out into a large shallow bowl or dish. Use a rice paddle or spatula and a slashing motion to spread the rice evenly in the bowl (don't toss; the rice can get gummy). Drizzle the rice vinegar over the rice. With the same slashing motion, mix until the grains are coated and glossy. Cover with a damp kitchen towel and cool at room temperature until cool enough to handle (do not refrigerate). Once cool, the rice will remain the right texture for making sushi for several hours.

Sassy Soups
AND STEWS

We like soup. There. We said it.
Don't think that makes us boring old farts.
These soups are really friggin' good. And
you can make a big batch and just heat it up for
dinner a few nights in a row. More time for sex!
Hah! Who's a boring old fart now, bitch?

Cheezy Cream of Broccoli

"Chicken" Noodle

Lentil Vegetable

Split Pea

Red Wine "Beef" Stew

Super Easy Creamy
"Chicken" and Gravy Stew

Cheezy Cream of Broccoli Soup

Makes about 7 cups

1 tablespoon refined coconut oil

1 onion, diced

4 cups roughly chopped
   broccoli florets

2 teaspoons fine sea salt

1 teaspoon pepper

1½ cups low-sodium
   vegetable stock

4 cups soy or rice milk

¼ cup arrowroot (or 5 tablespoons
   cornstarch) dissolved in ¼ cup
   cold water

6 ounces vegan cheddar cheese

So. Friggin'. Good.

Heat the coconut oil in a 4- to 6-quart stockpot over medium heat. Add the onion and cook, stirring occasionally, for 2 minutes. Add the broccoli, salt, and pepper and cook, stirring occasionally, until the onion is translucent and the broccoli is crisp-tender, about 4 minutes.

Stir in the stock, increase the heat to high, bring to a boil, and reduce the heat to a simmer. Cook until the broccoli is very tender, about 10 minutes. Remove from the heat and stir in about 1 cup of the soy or rice milk.

Transfer the mixture to a blender. On low or medium speed, puree until smooth. Transfer the mixture back to the pot, return to medium high heat, and stir in the remaining soy milk. When the soup returns to a simmer, add the arrowroot mixture and cheese, stirring until the cheese melts.

"Chicken" Noodle Soup

> Just like mom used to make—minus the pieces of decomposing, rotting chicken carcass.

Makes about 9 cups

1 tablespoon refined coconut oil

1 carrot, halved lengthwise and cut into ¼-inch slices

1 celery stalk, cut into ¼-inch slices

½ onion, cut into ½-inch dice

4 ounces white or cremini (brown) mushrooms, cut into ¼-inch slices

1 teaspoon fine sea salt

½ teaspoon pepper

¼ teaspoon curry powder

1 bay leaf

8 cups vegan chicken stock (hot water mixed with vegan chicken bouillon according to package directions)

2 teaspoons Bragg's Liquid Aminos (or 1¼ teaspoons tamari or soy sauce)

8 ounces vegan chicken strips or chunks (if frozen, no need to thaw)

4 ounces whole wheat or brown rice pasta

Heat the coconut oil in a 4- to 6-quart stockpot over medium heat. Add the carrot, celery, and onion and cook, stirring occasionally, until crisp tender, about 2 minutes. Add the mushrooms, salt, pepper, and curry powder and cook until the mushrooms release their juices, about 2 minutes.

Stir in the stock, Bragg's Liquid Aminos, and bay leaf. Increase the heat to high and bring to a boil. Add the chicken and pasta. When the soup returns to a boil, reduce to a simmer. Cook until the pasta is tender (time will depend on type of pasta). Remove the bay leaf and serve.

Lentil Vegetable Soup

Makes about 8 cups

1 tablespoon refined coconut oil

½ red bell pepper, cut into ½-inch dice

½ yellow bell pepper,
cut into ½-inch dice

½ onion, cut into ½-inch dice

1 zucchini, quartered lengthwise
and cut into ½-inch slices

1 yellow squash, quartered lengthwise and cut into ½-inch slices

4 cloves garlic, minced

1 teaspoon fine sea salt

½ teaspoon pepper

½ teaspoon dried marjoram

½ teaspoon dried thyme

⅛ teaspoon cayenne powder

6 cups low-sodium vegetable stock

1½ cups lentils

1 tablespoon tamari or soy sauce

½ teaspoon sesame oil

1 14.5-ounce can diced tomatoes
(with juices)

Heat the coconut oil in a 4- to 6-quart stockpot over medium heat. Add the red bell pepper, yellow bell pepper, and onion and cook, stirring occasionally, for 2 minutes. Add the zucchini, yellow squash, garlic, salt, pepper, marjoram, thyme, and cayenne and cook, stirring occasionally, for 1 minute.

Stir in the stock, lentils, and tamari or soy sauce. Increase the heat to high, bring to a boil, and reduce to a simmer. Cook until the lentils are tender, about 30 minutes. Add the sesame oil and tomatoes, stirring until the tomatoes are heated through.

WARNING: Lentils make you toot for hours. Plan accordingly.

Split Pea Soup

Makes about 8 cups

1 tablespoon refined
   coconut or safflower oil

8 strips vegan bacon,
   cut into ¼-inch dice

1 onion, cut into ¼-inch dice

4 cloves garlic, minced

1½ teaspoons dried oregano

1½ teaspoons fine sea salt

¾ teaspoon pepper

10 cups vegan chicken stock (hot
   water mixed with vegan chicken
   bouillon according to package
   directions)

3 cups split peas

1 carrot, cut into ¼-inch dice

1 celery stalk, cut into ¼-inch dice

Heat the oil in a 4- to 6-quart stockpot over medium, Add the bacon and cook, stirring occasionally, for 2 minutes. Add the onion and cook, stirring occasionally, for 1 minute. Add the garlic, oregano, salt, and pepper and cook, stirring occasionally, for 1 minute.

Stir in the stock and split peas. Increase the heat to high, bring to a boil, and reduce to a simmer. Cook for 45 minutes, stirring occasionally. Add the carrots and celery and cook, stirring occasionally, another 20 minutes, or until the carrots and celery are tender and the soup is the desired thickness.

Red Wine "Beef" Stew

Serves 6

½ cup whole wheat pastry flour

1 tablespoon minced fresh rosemary

1 teaspoon fine sea salt

½ teaspoon pepper

12 ounces vegan beef strips
    or chunks (thawed, if frozen)

1 tablespoon refined coconut oil

4 cloves garlic, minced

4½ cups low-sodium
    vegetable stock

1½ cups dry red wine

3 carrots, cut into 1-inch chunks

1 pound red potatoes, cut into
    1-inch chunks

1 onion, cut into 1-inch chunks

½ pounds cremini (brown) mush-
    rooms, halved (or quartered if large)

1 cup fresh or frozen peas

In a medium bowl, combine the flour, rosemary, salt, and pepper. Add the beef and toss to coat.

Heat the coconut oil in a 4- to 6-quart stockpot over medium heat. Add the beef mixture and cook, stirring occasionally, for 5 minutes. Add the garlic and cook, stirring occasionally, for 1 minute.

Stir in the stock, wine, and carrots. Increase the heat to high, bring to a boil, and reduce to a simmer. Cook for 15 minutes, stirring occasionally. Add the potato and onion and cook, stirring occasionally, for 15 minutes. Add the mushrooms and cook, stirring occasionally, for 15 minutes. Add the peas, stirring until the peas are heated through.

And you thought you needed a dead animal to make your stew hearty... Shame on you!

Super Easy Creamy "Chicken" and Gravy Stew

Serves 6

4 cups quadruple-strength vegan
  chicken stock (hot water mixed with
  four times the vegan chicken bouillon indicated on package directions)

1 (12-ounce) container vegan
  sour cream

¼ cup arrowroot or 5 tablespoons corn starch
  dissolved in ¼ cup water

¼ cup coarse nutritional yeast

2 teaspoons Bragg's Liquid Aminos (or
  1¼ teaspoons tamari or soy sauce)

1½ teaspoons garlic powder

1½ teaspoons onion powder

1 teaspoon dried tarragon

1 teaspoon fine sea salt

½ teaspoon pepper

½ teaspoon turmeric

16 ounces vegan chicken strips or
  chunks (if frozen, no need to thaw)

2 (14-ounce bags) frozen mixed
  vegetables, whatever vegetables
  you like — big chunks work best

In a 4- to 6-quart stockpot over medium high, combine the stock, sour cream, arrowroot mixture, nutritional yeast, Bragg's Liquid Aminos, garlic powder, onion powder, tarragon, salt, pepper, and turmeric, whisking until smooth. Bring the mixture to a simmer and stir in the chicken and vegetables. Return to a simmer and cook, stirring occasionally, until the chicken and vegetables are heated through (time will depend on the size of the chicken and vegetable pieces).

Skinny-Ass
SALADS

*Let's face it: Salads can be so fucking lame.
But they're really good for our bodies
(especially for pooping), so we gotta have 'em.
We crafted these little green monsters to be healthy
and yummy. This way, we don't have to suffer
through salads. We can actually enjoy them.*

Caesar Salad with
Homemade Herbed Croutons

Greek Salad

Chef's Salad

Tabouleh

Potato Salad with Fresh Dill

Edamame Three-bean Salad

Creamy Cole Slaw

Mediterranean Pasta Salad

Caesar Salad with Homemade Herbed Croutons

Serves 6 as an entree

or 8 to 10 as an appetizer

3 slices vegan whole wheat
  bread, diced

2 tablespoons refined coconut oil,
  melted, or safflower oil

1 teaspoon herbes de Provence
  (see note)

½ teaspoon fine sea salt

3 heads romaine lettuce,
  cut or torn into bite-sized pieces

About 1½ cups Vegan Caesar
  Dressing (see page 154)

Preheat oven to 375°F.

In a large bowl, combine the bread and oil. Stir in the herbes de Provence and salt. Spread the mixture onto a rimmed baking sheet and bake for 10 minutes. Remove from the oven and toss. Bake for 5 minutes more, or until browned. Cool the croutons thoroughly before using (or storing in an airtight container for up to 1 week).

In a large bowl, combine the romaine with the Vegan Caesar Dressing to taste. Toss in the croutons and serve.

> **HERBES de PROVENCE** is a dried herb blend. If you can't find it at your supermarket, try a specialty food store or substitute dried sage, thyme, rosemary, marjoram, or a combination.

Greek Salad

Serves 6 to 8 as a side dish
or 4 as an entree

2 tablespoons red wine vinegar

4 garlic cloves, minced

1 teaspoon Dijon mustard

½ teaspoon fine sea salt

½ teaspoon pepper

¼ cup extra virgin olive oil

2 tomatoes, cut into ¾-inch dice

1 cucumber, peeled, halved lengthwise, and cut into ¼-inch slices

½ cup pitted black olives,
   preferably Kalamata

¼ red onion, thinly sliced

3 cups Marinated Tofu "Feta"
   (see page 159)

Salad greens (optional)

In a small bowl, whisk together the red wine vinegar, garlic, mustard, salt, and pepper. Slowly whisk in the olive oil; set the dressing aside.

In a large bowl, combine the tomatoes, cucumber, olives, and onion. Gently toss in the Marinated Tofu "Feta" and dressing to taste. Serve as is for a side dish, or on top of salad greens for an entree.

Skinny-Ass Salads   63

Chef's Salad

Serves 4 as an entree

1 head red leaf, green leaf, or
   iceberg lettuce, torn into
   bite-sized pieces

4 slices vegan cheddar cheese,
   cut into strips

4 slices vegan Swiss or American
   cheese, cut into strips

4 slices vegan ham, cut into strips

4 slices vegan turkey, cut into strips

4 Roma tomatoes, cut into wedges

½ to 1 cup salad dressing of your
   choice (For Ranch see page 151,
   Thousand Island page 152,
   Caesar page 154)

1¼ cups "Egg" Salad (see page 44)

2 tablespoons chopped Italian
   parsley, for garnish (optional)

Arrange the lettuce on 4 plates, dividing it evenly. Artfully arrange the cheeses, ham, turkey, and tomatoes on top, dividing them evenly. Drizzle the salad dressing over the salads. Top with "Egg" Salad, dividing it evenly, and sprinkle with parsley, if using. Serve immediately.

Tabouleh

Serves 6 to 8

¾ cup bulgur wheat (see note)

1 cup boiling water

¼ cup extra virgin olive oil

1½ tablespoons lemon juice

½ teaspoon fine sea salt

¼ teaspoon pepper

1 tomato, cut into ½-inch dice

½ cucumber, peeled and cut
into ½-inch dice

¼ red onion, cut into ½-inch dice

⅓ cup roughly chopped fresh parsley

⅓ cup roughly chopped fresh mint

In a large bowl, combine the bulgur wheat and boiling water. Cover and set aside for 30 minutes. Meanwhile, in a small bowl, combine the olive oil, lemon juice, salt, and pepper; set aside.

Add the tomato, cucumber, and onion to the bulgur wheat. Stir in the parsley and mint. Add the dressing and toss gently.

BULGUR WHEAT can be found in the bulk section of many major supermarkets as well as at natural food stores.

Potato Salad with Fresh Dill

Serves 6 to 8

6 cups water

1½ pounds red or Yukon gold
potatoes, cut into 1-inch cubes

About 2½ teaspoons fine sea salt

⅓ cup vegan mayonnaise

¼ cup sweet pickle relish

1 teaspoon white wine vinegar

¼ teaspoon pepper

1 celery stalk, cut into ½-inch dice
or thinly sliced

2 scallions, thinly sliced

2 tablespoons chopped fresh dill

In a 3- or 4-quart stockpot, combine the water with about 2 teaspoons of the salt. Add the potatoes and place the pot over high heat. Bring to a boil, reduce to a simmer, and cook until the potatoes are tender, about 5 minutes. Strain the potatoes and transfer them to a large bowl to cool.

Meanwhile, in a small bowl, whisk together the mayonnaise, pickle relish, vinegar, pepper, and remaining ½ teaspoon of salt.

When the potatoes are cool, gently toss in the celery, scallions, and dill. Add the mayonnaise mixture and gently toss.

Edamame Three-bean Salad

Serves 6 to 8

2 tablespoons red wine vinegar

1 teaspoon Dijon mustard

½ teaspoon fine sea salt

¼ teaspoon pepper

3 tablespoons extra virgin olive oil

1 ear corn or ½ cup frozen corn
   (rinsed under cold water to thaw)

1 cup shelled soy beans (edamame)
   (see note)

1 (15- to 16-ounce) can red kidney
   beans, drained and rinsed

1 (15- to 16-ounce) can garbanzo
   beans, drained and rinsed

2 scallions, cut into ½-inch slices

½ red bell pepper,
   cut into ½-inch dice

2 tablespoons chopped fresh
   Italian parsley

2 tablespoons chopped fresh
   cilantro, basil, or a combination

In a small bowl, whisk together the red wine vinegar, mustard, salt, and pepper. Slowly whisk in the olive oil; set aside.

Cut the kernels off the ear of corn and place them in a large bowl. Stir in the soy beans, kidney beans, garbanzo beans, scallions, bell pepper, parsley, and cilantro and/or basil. Gently toss in the dressing.

> **SHELLED SOY BEANS,** also known as edamame, can be found in the produce or freezer section of many major supermarkets, as well as at natural and Asian food stores. If frozen, rinse under cold water to thaw.

Creamy Cole Slaw

Serves 4 to 6

¼ cup vegan mayonnaise

¼ cup vegan sour cream

½ tablespoon white wine vinegar

½ tablespoon agave nectar

½ teaspoon fine sea salt

½ head green cabbage, quartered, cored, and thinly shredded

⅛ small red cabbage, halved, cored and thinly shredded

1 carrot, shredded

In a small bowl, whisk together the mayonnaise, sour cream, vinegar, agave nectar, and salt; set aside.

In a large bowl, combine the green cabbage, red cabbage, and carrot. Add the dressing and toss until well combined. Cover and refrigerate for 24 to 48 hours to let the flavors develop.

Lazy bitches can replace the green cabbage, red cabbage, and carrot with a one-pound bag of prepared slaw mix.

Mediterranean Pasta Salad

Serves 10 to 12

3 quarts water

About 1½ tablespoons fine sea salt

1 pound whole wheat fusilli, rotelli,
   or other shaped pasta

½ cup oil-packed julienned
   sun-dried tomatoes, drained
   (save 2 tablespoons of oil)

1 lemon

1 (14.75-ounce) jar marinated
   artichoke hearts, drained (save
   2 tablespoons of marinade)

½ cup pitted black olives (Kalamata,
   Niçoise — anything other than
   canned Mission olives)

½ cup chopped fresh basil

In a 4- to 6-quart stockpot over high heat, combine the water and salt. Bring the water to a boil, add the pasta, and cook according to the package directions. When the pasta is done, drain it (don't rinse it), transfer it to a large bowl, and toss with the 2 tablespoons of reserved sun dried tomato oil. Set aside to cool.

Meanwhile, juice the lemon into a small bowl. Whisk in the 2 tablespoons of artichoke marinade. Set aside.

When the pasta is cool, gently toss in the marinade mixture. Cut the artichoke pieces in half (or quarters if large) and add them to the pasta, along with the sun-dried tomatoes, olives, and basil. Gently toss to combine. Serve immediately or refrigerate until serving.

Hearty-Ass
SANDWICHES

*The only thing better than pigging out on
a big-ass sandwich? Getting seconds from off
your own face. Moo! Chow down, cowgirls!*

Club Sandwich

Reuben-esque

"Tuna" Salad

"Chicken" Salad

Philly "Cheesesteak"

Veggie Burger

"Chicken" Panini

Club Sandwich

Makes 4 sandwiches

8 slices vegan whole wheat
   bread, toasted

About 3 tablespoons
   vegan mayonnaise

1 avocado, sliced

8 ounces vegan turkey
   or chicken slices

2 tomatoes, sliced

12 strips vegan bacon

4 large lettuce leaves

Spread each slice of toast with about 2 teaspoons of the mayonnaise. Top the mayonnaise side with 4 slices with avocado, turkey or chicken, tomatoes, bacon, and lettuce, dividing the ingredients evenly. Top with remaining toast, mayonnaise side down.

Reuben-esque

Makes 1 sandwich

¼ cup low-sodium vegetable stock

1 teaspoon garlic powder

½ teaspoon Bragg's Liquid Aminos
  (or ¼ teaspoon tamari or soy sauce)

6 to 12 strips vegan bacon

2 slices vegan whole wheat rye
  bread, toasted

2 slices vegan Swiss cheese

¼ cup drained sauerkraut

2 tablespoons Thousand Island
  Dressing (see page 152)

Preheat broiler.

In a 12-inch nonstick skillet over medium heat, combine the stock, garlic powder, and Bragg's Liquid Aminos. When the mixture begins simmering, add the bacon strips, spreading them out evenly. Cook until the liquid has evaporated, about 2 minutes. Turn and cook the other side until the garlic powder begins to brown, about 1 minute.

Remove from heat; set aside.

Arrange the bacon on top of one slice of toast. Top with the cheese and place on a baking sheet. Arrange the sauerkraut on the other slice of toast and place on the baking sheet. Place the baking sheet under the broiler until the cheese melts and the sauerkraut is warm. (Time will depend on the cheese. Keep a watchful eye on it! It could only take a minute or so.) Remove from the broiler, top sauerkraut with Thousand Island Dressing, and sandwich the two toasts together. Cut in half and serve.

FYI: Six slices of bacon strips make for a satisfying sandwich; twelve make for a whaler. For the complete deli experience, hold the sandwich together with toothpicks and serve a sour pickle on the side.

Hearty-Ass Sandwiches   73

"Tuna" Salad Sandwich

Makes 3 or 4 sandwiches

2 cups finely shredded parsnip

1 celery stalk, finely diced

¼ small red or white onion,
   finely diced

1 lemon

¼ cup vegan mayonnaise

½ tablespoon sweet pickle relish

1 teaspoon coarse nutritional yeast

½ teaspoon kelp powder

¼ teaspoon fine sea salt

6 to 8 slices vegan
   whole wheat bread

In a large bowl, combine the parsnip, celery, and onion. Zest, then halve the lemon. Add the lemon zest and juice from one half (save the other for another use) to the parsnip mixture, along with the mayonnaise, relish, yeast, kelp powder, and salt, stirring to combine.

Spread the tuna salad on 3 or 4 slices of bread, top with remaining 3 or 4 slices, and serve.

"Chicken" Salad Sandwich

Makes 3 or 4 sandwiches

½ cup vegan mayonnaise

2 teaspoons lemon juice

1 tablespoon coarse nutritional yeast

½ tablespoon agave nectar

¼ teaspoon fine sea salt

¼ teaspoon curry powder

⅛ teaspoon pepper

2 cups chopped or shredded vegan
  chicken strips or chunks (thawed,
  if frozen)

¼ cup halved (quartered if large)
  seedless red grapes (optional)

1 celery stalk, finely diced

¼ small red or white onion,
  finely diced

2 tablespoons chopped fresh
  Italian parsley

6 to 8 slices vegan
  whole wheat bread

In a small bowl, combine the mayonnaise, lemon juice, yeast, agave nectar, salt, curry powder, and pepper. In a large bowl, combine the chicken, grapes (if using), celery, onion, and parsley. Add the mayonnaise mixture to the chicken mixture, tossing gently.

Spread the chicken salad on 3 or 4 slices of bread, top with remaining 3 or 4 slices, and serve.

> If you're one of those lunatics who doesn't eat bread, you can also serve this salad on a bed of lettuce.

Philly "Cheesesteak"

Makes 2 sandwiches

2 tablespoons refined coconut oil

½ red bell pepper,
    cut into ¼-inch slices

½ yellow or green bell pepper, cut
    into ¼-inch slices

½ red onion, cut into ¼-inch slices

4 ounces brown or white
    mushrooms, sliced

2 cloves garlic, minced

½ teaspoon fine sea salt

¼ teaspoon pepper

12 slices vegan bacon

About ¼ cup water

4 slices vegan American cheese

2 vegan soft whole wheat rolls

Heat the coconut oil in a 10- to 12-inch skillet over medium heat. Add the peppers and cook, stirring occasionally, for 5 minutes. Add the onion and cook, stirring occasionally, until onion is lightly browned, about 3 minutes. Add the mushrooms and cook, stirring occasionally, for 3 minutes more. Add the garlic, reduce the heat to low, and cook, stirring occasionally, until all the vegetables are very tender, 5 to 7 minutes. Remove from the heat and stir in the salt and pepper. Transfer to a bowl, cover with a dish or plastic wrap, and set aside to steam.

Return the skillet to medium heat and add about 2 tablespoons of water. Use a spatula to loosen any caramelized bits in the skillet, then add the bacon (it can overlap slightly, but you may have to do two batches). Cook about 2 minutes, turning once. If the skillet gets dry, add more water, 1 tablespoon at a time (you want the bacon tender and juicy, not crisp).

Cut the rolls almost in half lengthwise, then gently fold each open. Pile 6 strips of bacon, 2 slices of cheese, and half of the veggies onto each of the rolls.

Veggie Burger Four Ways

Funny how we associate being "All-American" with eating the flesh of a tortured, slaughtered animal... Well, not in Skinny Bitch world!

ALL-AMERICAN BASIC BURGER

Makes 4 burgers

4 vegan burger patties

4 slices vegan cheese (optional)

4 large lettuce leaves

1 large tomato,
   cut into 4 thick slices

4 thin slices red onion

12 slices "bread and butter" pickles

4 vegan whole wheat hamburger
   buns, split and toasted

Mustard, ketchup, and vegan
   mayonnaise, for serving

Grill or pan-sauté the burger patties according to package directions. If using cheese, top each patty with one slice of cheese during the last minute of cooking.

Meanwhile, arrange lettuce, tomato, red onion, and pickles on serving plates, dividing evenly. When the patties are done, sandwich one between each bun, arrange on plates, and serve.

PIZZA BURGER

Makes 4 burgers

4 vegan burger patties

4 slices vegan mozzarella cheese

16 slices vegan pepperoni

4 vegan whole wheat hamburger
buns, split and toasted

¾ cup Pizza Sauce (see page 157),
warmed

12 large basil leaves,
cut into thin strips

Pan-sauté the burger patties according to package directions. Top each patty with one slice of cheese during the last minute of cooking. Add the pepperoni to the pan during the last minute as well, just to warm it.

Place one cooked patty on the bottom of each bun. Top with Pizza Sauce, pepperoni, and basil leaves, dividing evenly. Serve immediately.

....

CALIFORNIA BURGER

Makes 4 burgers

4 vegan burger patties

4 vegan whole wheat hamburger
buns, split and toasted

1 avocado, sliced

1 cup loosely packed alfalfa sprouts

½ cup Thousand Island Dressing
(see page 152)

Grill or pan-sauté the burger patties according to package directions. Place one cooked patty on the bottom of each bun. Top with avocado, sprouts, and Thousand Island Dressing, dividing evenly. Serve immediately.

BACON AND CARAMELIZED ONION CHEESEBURGERS WITH AGAVE-DIJON

Makes 4 burgers

¼ cup refined coconut oil

2 large yellow onions,
   cut into ¼-inch slices

¼ teaspoon fine sea salt

⅛ teaspoon pepper

2 tablespoons agave nectar

2 tablespoons Dijon mustard

8 slices vegan bacon

4 vegan burger patties

4 slices vegan cheese

4 vegan whole wheat hamburger
   buns, split and toasted

Heat the coconut oil in a large skillet over medium-high heat. Add the onions and cook, stirring occasionally, until translucent, about 5 minutes. Reduce the heat to very low and cook, stirring occasionally, until the onions are deeply golden, about 45 minutes. Stir in the salt and pepper and set aside to cool.

While the onions are cooking, whisk together the agave and mustard in a small bowl; set aside.

While the onions are cooling, cook the bacon according to package directions. Grill or pan-sauté the burger patties according to package directions. Top each patty with one slice of cheese during the last minute of cooking. Place one cooked patty on the bottom of each bun. Top with onions, bacon, and mustard mixture, dividing evenly. Serve immediately.

Grilled "Chicken" Panini Three Ways

"CHICKEN" PARMESAN PANINI

Makes 4 panini

2 tablespoons refined coconut oil
(optional)

4 vegan soft whole wheat rolls or
8 slices vegan whole wheat bread

16 vegan chicken nuggets, cooked
according to package directions

1 cup Basic Red Sauce
(see page 156)

4 to 8 slices vegan
mozzarella cheese

Spread the coconut oil if using, on the top and bottom of the rolls or one side of each slice of bread, dividing it evenly. Cut open the rolls or lay the bread, oiled side down if applicable, on a work surface. Top the bottom half of the rolls or four slices of the bread with the chicken nuggets, Red Sauce, and cheese, dividing evenly.

In a large nonstick skillet over medium heat, cook two sandwiches, covered, about 4 minutes, until golden brown. Flip the sandwiches and cook, uncovered, until the second side is golden brown and the cheese has melted, about 2 minutes. Repeat with the remaining two sandwiches. (Alternately, cook the sandwiches on a panini grill until the bread is golden brown and the cheese has melted, 2 to 3 minutes.)

MEDITERRANEAN "CHICKEN" PANINI

Makes 4 panini

2 tablespoons refined coconut oil
  (optional)
4 vegan soft whole wheat rolls or
  8 slices vegan whole wheat bread
4 vegan chicken patties, cooked
  according to package directions
About 40 large basil leaves
1 cup roasted red pepper strips,
  drained
4 to 8 slices vegan mozzarella
  cheese

Spread the coconut oil, if using, on the top and bottom of the rolls or one side of each slice of bread, dividing it evenly. Cut open the rolls or lay the bread, oiled side down if applicable, on a work surface. Top the bottom half of the rolls or four slices of bread with the chicken, basil, peppers, and cheese, dividing evenly.

In a large nonstick skillet over medium heat, cook two sandwiches, covered, about 4 minutes, until golden brown. Flip the sandwiches and cook, uncovered, until the second side is golden brown and the cheese has melted, about 2 minutes. Repeat with the remaining two sandwiches. (Alternately, cook the sandwiches on a panini grill until the bread is golden brown and the cheese has melted, 2 to 3 minutes.)

BARBECUE "CHICKEN" PANINI

Makes 4 panini

2 tablespoons refined coconut oil
   (optional)
4 vegan soft whole wheat rolls or
   8 slices vegan whole wheat bread
¾ cup barbecue sauce
4 vegan chicken patties, cooked
   according to package directions
1 cup Creamy Cole Slaw
   (see page 68)

Spread the coconut oil, if using, on the top and bottom of the rolls or one side of each slice of bread, dividing it evenly. Cut open the rolls or lay the bread, buttered side down if applicable, on a work surface. Top the bottom half of the rolls or four slices of the bread with the barbecue sauce, chicken, and Creamy Cole Slaw, dividing evenly.

In a large nonstick skillet over medium heat, cook two sandwiches, covered, about 4 minutes, until golden brown. Flip the sandwiches and cook, uncovered, until the second side is golden brown, about 2 minutes. Repeat with the remaining two sandwiches. (Alternately, cook the sandwiches on a panini grill until the bread is golden brown, 2 to 3 minutes.)

International BITCH

You can totally pretend to be cooler
and worldlier than you actually are.
Just make one of these global goodies.

Falafel

Japanese Soba Noodles
with Steamed Vegetables and Tofu

Potato and Pumpkin Curry
with Brown Basmati Rice

Pad Thai

Veggie Enchiladas

Falafel

....

Makes 6 sandwiches

1 (15- to 16-ounce) can garbanzo
   beans, drained and rinsed

½ onion, coarsely chopped

2 tablespoons vegan whole wheat
   panko (Japanese bread crumbs)
   or whole wheat bread crumbs

2 tablespoons chickpea
   (garbanzo) flour or whole wheat
   pastry flour

2 tablespoons coarsely chopped
   Italian parsley

½ teaspoon ground cumin

½ teaspoon ground coriander

¼ teaspoon pepper

4 cloves garlic

½ to ¾ teaspoon fine sea salt,
   plus more for sprinkling

About 2 tablespoons refined
   coconut oil, melted, or safflower oil

1 lemon

6 tablespoons tahini

¼ cup water

3 tablespoons extra virgin olive oil

¼ teaspoon paprika

6 (6-inch) pita breads

¼ head iceberg, romaine,
   green leaf, or red leaf lettuce,
   coarsely shredded

1 tomato, cut into thin wedges

½ cucumber, cut into ¼-inch slices

12 to 18 slices dill pickle

Preheat oven to 350°F.

In a food processor, combine the garbanzo beans, onion, panko, flour, parsley, cumin, coriander, pepper, 2 cloves of the garlic, and ½ teaspoon of the salt. Pulse, scraping the sides of the bowl as necessary, to form a coarse paste. Shape the paste into 12 to 14 golf ball-sized rounds. Flatten the balls to about ¾-inch thick and transfer to a rimmed baking sheet. Brush both sides of each ball with the coconut or safflower oil and bake for 45 minutes, turning halfway through, until nicely browned. Set aside to cool.

Meanwhile, juice the lemon. In a small bowl, whisk together the tahini, water, olive oil, paprika, lemon juice, and ¼ teaspoon salt (if using unsalted tahini). Press or finely mince the remaining 2 cloves of garlic and whisk into the tahini sauce. Set aside until ready to serve, or refrigerate for up to a week.

To assemble the sandwiches, cut about 1-inch off the top of each pita, forming a pocket. Add falafel, lettuce, tomato, cucumber, and pickle, dividing evenly. Drizzle each sandwich with about a tablespoon of tahini and pass the rest at the table.

International Bitch 87

Japanese Soba Noodles with Steamed Vegetables and Tofu

Serves 3 or 4

2 tablespoons mirin (see note)

1 tablespoon minced fresh ginger

1 tablespoon tamari or soy sauce

2 teaspoons sesame oil

¼ cup seasoned rice vinegar

½ pound globe eggplant, cut into ½-inch cubes, or Chinese or Japanese eggplant, cut into ¼-inch slices

About 4¾ teaspoons fine sea salt

8 ounces firm or extra firm tofu, cut into ¼-inch cubes

1 carrot, cut into matchsticks

8 ounces buckwheat soba noodles

3 scallions, thinly sliced

1 tablespoon gomasio (see note) or toasted sesame seeds

In a large bowl, whisk together the mirin, ginger, tamari or soy sauce, and 1 teaspoon of the sesame oil; set aside.

In a pot fitted with a steamer insert, bring 1 inch of water and 2 tablespoons of the rice vinegar to a boil. Arrange the eggplant in the insert, sprinkle with ¼ teaspoon salt, cover, and steam for 7 minutes. Add the carrot and steam for 5 to 8 minutes. Add the tofu and steam for 3 minutes, until the vegetables are tender and the tofu is heated through.

Meanwhile, in a 4- to 6-quart stockpot, combine 3 quarts of water with about 1½ tablespoons salt. Bring to a boil over high heat, add the noodles, and cook according to package directions until tender. Drain, rinse in cold water, drain again, and return the noodles to the pot. Toss with the remaining 1 teaspoon of sesame oil and cover.

When the vegetable mixture is cooked, add it to the bowl with the mirin mixture, tossing gently.

To serve, place the noodles on plates or a platter and top with the vegetable mixture, scallions, and gomasio, dividing evenly. Serve hot or room temperature.

MIRIN (Japanese rice wine used for cooking) can be found at Asian markets and in the international section of many supermarkets.

GOMASIO is a seasoning made of sesame seeds, seaweed, and sea salt. You can find it at Asian markets and some health food stores.

Potato and Pumpkin Curry with Brown Basmati Rice

Serves 4 to 6

1½ cups brown basmati rice

2½ cups water

¾ teaspoon fine sea salt, divided

2 tablespoons refined coconut oil

1 onion, cut into ¾-inch chunks

2 cloves garlic, minced

1 (14.5-ounce) can diced tomatoes
   (with juices)

1 cup low-sodium vegetable stock

1 teaspoon ground cumin

1 teaspoon ground coriander

½ teaspoon turmeric

⅛ teaspoon cayenne

⅛ teaspoon ground cinnamon

⅛ teaspoon ground cloves

1 pound red potatoes,
   cut into ¾-inch chunks

3 cups ¾-inch chunks pumpkin
   (see note)

1½ tablespoons lemon juice

1 tablespoon chopped fresh
   cilantro or Italian parsley

In a 2-quart saucepan over high heat, combine the rice, water, and ¼ teaspoon of the salt. Bring to a boil, reduce the heat to a simmer, cover, and cook until the water is absorbed and the rice is tender, about 30 minutes. Remove from the heat and let the rice stand, covered, at least 10 minutes.

While the rice is standing, make the curry: Heat the coconut oil in a 10- to 12-inch skillet over medium high. Add the onion and cook, stirring occasionally, until almost tender, about 3 minutes. Stir in the garlic and cook 1 minute more. Add the tomatoes, stock, cumin, coriander, turmeric, cayenne, cinnamon, cloves, and remaining ½ teaspoon of salt.

Bring to a boil and add the potatoes and pumpkin. Return to a boil, reduce to a simmer, cover, and cook, stirring occasionally, until the potato and pumpkin are tender, about 15 minutes. Remove from heat and stir in lemon juice.

Serve over rice sprinkled with cilantro.

Pumpkin doesn't have to be peeled or skinned before cooking. If you can't find pumpkin, substitute butternut squash, which does have to be skinned. A vegetable peeler works well.

Pad Thai

Serves 3 to 4

6 ounces rice stick noodles

¼ cup agave nectar

¼ cup mirin (see note page 89)

3 tablespoons ketchup

3 tablespoons tamari or soy sauce

1½ tablespoons lime juice

1 tablespoon sriracha (see note
   page 49) or other chili sauce

2 tablespoons refined coconut oil

14 to 16 ounces extra-firm tofu,
   cubed

½ red onion, cut into ¼-inch slices

2 cloves garlic, minced

3 scallions, halved lengthwise and
   cut into 2-inch pieces

2 cups bean sprouts

1 carrot, shredded

¼ cup chopped fresh cilantro, mint,
   or a combination

¼ cup chopped roasted peanuts

4 to 8 lime wedges

Cook the noodles according to package directions. Drain and set aside.

Meanwhile, in a small bowl, whisk together the agave, mirin, ketchup, tamari or soy sauce, lime juice, and sriracha; set aside.

Heat the coconut oil in a 12- to 14-inch wok or skillet over high. Add the tofu and stir-fry for 4 minutes. Add the red onion and stir-fry for 30 seconds. Add the garlic and stir-fry for 30 seconds. Add the noodles and agave nectar mixture and stir-fry until the noodles are softened and evenly coated with sauce. Add the scallions, bean sprouts, and carrot and stir-fry until all the ingredients are well combined and heated through.

Transfer the pad thai to plates or a platter, garnish with cilantro or mint, peanuts and lime wedges, and serve.

> We know it seems like the ketchup would crap up the whole dish, but it doesn't. Trust your Bitches.

Veggie Enchiladas

Serves 6

2 tablespoons refined coconut or safflower oil, plus more for frying

1 red bell pepper, cut into ½-inch dice

1 yellow or green bell pepper, cut into ½-inch dice

1 red onion, cut into ½-inch dice

2 cloves garlic, minced

3 cups enchilada sauce, homemade (recipe follows) or canned

1 cup fresh corn, cooked, or frozen corn, thawed

1 (2¼-ounce) can sliced Mission olives, drained

1 teaspoon fine sea salt

½ teaspoon ground cumin

½ teaspoon ground coriander

12 (7-inch) corn tortillas

4 ounces vegan cheddar cheese, shredded

2 scallions, thinly sliced

Preheat oven to 350°F.

Heat 2 tablespoons of the oil in a 10- to 12-inch skillet over medium heat. Add the bell peppers and cook, stirring occasionally, for 5 minutes. Add the onion and cook, stirring occasionally, for 5 minutes. Add the garlic, reduce the heat to low, and cook, stirring occasionally, until all the vegetables are very tender, about 10 minutes. Transfer the vegetables to a large bowl and stir in ½ cup of the enchilada sauce, the corn, olives, salt, cumin, and coriander.

Warm the remaining enchilada sauce in a small saucepan. Then transfer the sauce to a round 8- or 9-inch cake pan. Working one tortilla at a time, use tongs to dip the tortilla into the warm enchilada sauce, dipping to soften the tortilla and coat both sides. Transfer the tortilla to a plate and spoon about ¼ cup of the vegetable mixture down the center of the tortilla. Roll the tortilla into a tight cylinder, enclosing the filling. Transfer

International Bitch   93

the filled tortilla to a 13 x 9-inch baking pan, seam side down. Repeat with remaining tortillas, making 2 rows of 6 enchiladas each in the baking pan.

Pour the leftover dipping sauce over the enchiladas, covering them evenly.

Sprinkle the cheese over the sauce. Bake for 20 minutes, or until the tip of a knife inserted into the center of an enchilada comes out piping hot. Sprinkle with scallions and serve.

ENCHILADA SAUCE

Makes about 3 cups

10 dried California or other
  mild chiles, stemmed,
  split, and seeds removed

5 cups water

1 clove garlic

¼ cup refined coconut oil,
  melted, or safflower oil

1 tablespoon tomato paste

1 teaspoon ground cumin

1 teaspoon dried oregano

1 teaspoon fine sea salt

In a 10- to 12-inch skillet over medium high heat, toast the chiles a few at a time until they're blistered and a few shades darker, 1 to 1½ minutes, turning occasionally. Transfer to a bowl and cover with the water. Place a plate on top of the chiles to keep them submerged in the water (if necessary, place something heavy, like a can or two, on top of the plate). Set aside for 30 minutes.

Drain off 2 cups of the water. Place the chiles and remaining water in a blender, along with the garlic, oil, tomato paste, cumin, oregano, and salt. Puree until smooth. Transfer the mixture to a 2- or 3-quart saucepan over high heat. Bring to a boil, reduce to a simmer, and cook 10 minutes.

Italian
BITCH

Oh, Italian food, how we love thee.
When everyone was forsaking you for
"low carb" diets, we never turned our backs on you.
And we never will, Italian food. We never will.

East Coast Lasagna

Stuffed Shells

Penne with Butternut Squash,
Sage Pesto, and Almonds

Fettuccine Alfredo

Linguini with Pesto, Pine Nuts,
and Sun-dried Tomatoes

Eggplant Parmesan

East Coast Lasagna

Serves 8 to 12

6 quarts water

About 3 tablespoons fine sea salt

1 pound whole wheat or brown rice
  lasagna noodles

5 cups Basic Red Sauce
  (see page 156)

4 cups Tofu "Ricotta" (see page 158)

12 to 14 ounces vegan ground beef
  (if frozen, no need to thaw)

10 ounces vegan mozzarella
  cheese, shredded

Preheat oven to 350°F.

In an 8- to 10-quart stockpot over high heat, combine the water with about 3 tablespoons salt. Bring the water to a boil, add the lasagna noodles, and cook according to the package directions. When the pasta is done, drain it, briefly rinse it (just to make it cool enough to handle), and drain it again. Separate the noodles and lay them on foil, waxed paper, or parchment paper to keep them from sticking together.

Spread ½ cup of the Basic Red sauce in the bottom of a 13 x 9-inch pan. Top the sauce with some of the lasagna noodles, overlapping them slightly. Top the noodles with ⅓ of the Tofu Ricotta, ⅓ of the ground beef, and ⅓ of the cheese, spreading each layer of ingredients out evenly. Repeat the noodles, Tofu Ricotta, ground beef, and cheese layers two more times (you may not need all of the pasta).

Place the pan of lasagna on a rimmed baking sheet and bake until the tip of a knife inserted in the center of the lasagna comes out piping hot, 60 to 75 minutes. (Check on it periodically to make sure the cheese isn't burning. If it seems like it might, cover with foil until the final 15 minutes.) Remove the lasagna from the oven and let it sit 10 to 15 minutes before cutting and serving. Then chow the hell down!

Stuffed Shells with Red or White Sauce

Makes 22 to 24 shells,

to serve 6 to 8

3 quarts water

About 5 teaspoons fine sea salt

8 ounces whole wheat or brown rice
jumbo pasta shells

1 tablespoon refined coconut oil

½ onion, finely diced

2 cloves garlic, minced

2 cups Tofu "Ricotta"
(see page 158)

1 (10-ounce) package frozen
chopped spinach, thawed and
squeezed of excess water

2 tablespoons vegan Parmesan
cheese

2 tablespoons whole
wheat bread crumbs

¼ teaspoon pepper

2 cups Basic Red Sauce (see
page 156) or Savory White
Cream Sauce (see page 148)

Preheat oven to 350°F.

In a 4- to 6-quart stockpot over high heat, combine the water with about 1½ tablespoons of the salt. Bring the water to a boil, add the shells, and cook according to the package directions. When the pasta is done, drain it, briefly rinse it (just to make it cool enough to handle), and drain it again.

Meanwhile, heat the coconut oil in an 8- to 10-inch skillet over medium. Add the onions and cook, stirring occasionally, until tender, 4 to 6 minutes. Stir in the garlic and cook, stirring occasionally, 1 minute. Transfer the onion mixture to a large bowl and mix in the remaining ½ teaspoon salt, along with the Tofu Ricotta, spinach, cheese, bread crumbs, and pepper.

Spread about 1 cup of the Basic Red Sauce or Savory White Cream Sauce in the bottom of a 13 x 9-inch pan. Stuff each shell with about 2 tablespoons of the Tofu Ricotta mixture, arranging the stuffed shells on top of the sauce (you may not need all of the shells). Top each shell with a dollop of the remaining sauce, dividing it evenly. Cover the pan with foil and bake until the tip of a knife inserted in the center of one of the shells comes out piping hot, about 30 minutes.

> Stuffed friggin' shells! Vegan style! Could you die or what?

Penne with Butternut Squash, Sage Pesto, and Almonds

Serves 4

3 quarts water

About 5 teaspoons fine sea salt

8 ounces whole wheat or
   brown rice penne

2 tablespoons refined coconut oil

1½ pounds butternut squash,
   peeled, seeded, and cut into
   ¼ inch thick sticks

2 shallots, thinly sliced

¼ teaspoon pepper

½ cup Sage Pesto (see page 155)

¼ cup sliced almonds,
   toasted (optional)

In a 4- to 6-quart stockpot over high heat, combine the water with about 1½ tablespoons salt. Bring the water to a boil, add the penne, and cook according to the package directions.

Meanwhile, heat the coconut oil in a 10- to 12-inch skillet over medium-high heat. Add the squash and cook, stirring occasionally, for 4 minutes. Stir in the shallots, pepper, and the remaining ½ teaspoon salt and cook, stirring occasionally, until the squash and shallots are tender, 1 to 2 minutes. Remove from the heat and set aside.

When the pasta is done, drain it, reserving ½ cup of the pasta cooking water. Return the pasta to the pot and stir in the pesto and the squash mixture. If it seems too dry, add ¼ to ½ cup of the pasta water. Transfer the pasta to plates or a platter, and if desired, garnish with almonds. Serve immediately.

Fettuccini Alfredo

Serves 3 to 4

3 quarts water

About 4¾ teaspoons fine sea salt

8 ounces whole wheat or brown rice
fettuccini

¼ cup refined coconut oil

½ cup vegan creamer

¼ cup vegan Parmesan cheese

¼ teaspoon pepper

2 cups fresh peas, cooked, or
frozen peas, thawed (optional)

In a 4- to 6-quart stockpot over high heat, combine the water with about 1½ tablespoons salt. Bring the water to a boil, add the fettuccini, and cook according to the package directions.

Meanwhile, in a 1- to 2-quart saucepan over medium heat, melt the coconut oil. When it's almost melted, whisk in the creamer, increase the heat to medium high, and bring to a simmer. Whisk in the Parmesan, pepper, and the remaining ¼ teaspoon of salt. Cover and set aside.

When the pasta is done, drain it, reserving ½ cup of the pasta cooking water. Return the pasta to the pot and stir in the sauce (re-whisk if it separated) and peas, if using. If it seems too dry, add ¼ to ½ cup of the pasta water. Transfer the pasta to plates or a platter and serve.

Linguini with Pesto, Pine Nuts, and Sun-dried Tomatoes

Serves 3 to 4

3 quarts water

About 1½ tablespoons fine sea salt

8 ounces whole wheat or
  brown rice linguini

½ cup Basil Pesto (see page 155)

½ cup oil-packed julienned
  sun-dried tomatoes, drained

½ cup pine nuts, toasted, divided

Zest of 1 lemon (optional)

¼ cup roughly chopped
  fresh basil leaves

In a 4- to 6-quart stockpot over high heat, combine the water with about 1½ tablespoons salt. Bring the water to a boil, add the linguini, and cook according to the package directions. When the pasta is done, drain it, reserving ½ cup of the pasta cooking water.

Return the pasta to the pot and stir in the pesto, sun-dried tomatoes, about ¾ of the pine nuts, and the lemon zest, if using. If the pasta seems too dry, add ¼ to ½ cup of the pasta water. Transfer the pasta to plates or a platter, garnish with the basil leaves and remaining pine nuts, and serve.

Eggplant Parmesan

If you're one of those baby bitches— "I don't like eggplant"—now is the time to get over it.

Serves 4 as an entree

or 8 as a side dish or appetizer

¾ cup vegan Parmesan cheese

⅓ cup whole wheat bread crumbs

1 tablespoon granulated garlic powder

2 teaspoons fine sea salt

¾ teaspoon pepper

½ cup soy or rice milk

Refined coconut oil

1 eggplant (about 1½ pounds), cut crosswise into ½-inch slices

1½ cups Basic Red Sauce (see page 156)

¼ cup roughly chopped fresh basil leaves

4 ounces vegan mozzarella cheese, shredded

Preheat oven to 350°F.

In a shallow bowl, combine the Parmesan, bread crumbs, garlic powder, salt, and pepper. Place the soy or rice milk in another shallow bowl. Heat 3 to 4 tablespoons of oil, enough to coat the pan with a thin layer in a 10- or 12-inch nonstick skillet over medium.

One at a time, dip the eggplant slices in the soy or rice milk, then the bread-crumb mixture, pressing to thoroughly coat. Place the finished slices in the hot pan and cook about 3 minutes per side, or until browned on the outside and tender on the inside (you'll have to do more than one batch; wipe out the pan between batches and add more oil). Transfer the finished slices to a 2-quart casserole dish, arranging them into two layers. Top the eggplant with the sauce, spreading it evenly. Top the sauce with the basil and mozzarella, sprinkling both evenly. Bake until the sauce is hot and cheese is melted, about 20 minutes.

Down Home COOKIN'

If the shoe fits, wear it. And if you like to eat shit,
eat it. And don't feel bad about it, neither.
Here are a few old favorites that you might ordinarily
feel guilty about eating. But now you can indulge
without feeling fat or sick. (You can send us
"thank-you" notes via www.SkinnyBitch.net.)

Macaroni and Four Cheeses

Oven-fried "Chicken" and Cornbread

Cha Cha Chili

Potatoes au Gratin

Shepherd's Pie

Cheezy Casserole

"Meatloaf" with Mashed Potatoes and Gravy

Sloppy Joes

Potato Skins with all the Fixin's

Macaroni and Four Cheeses

Serves 8

1 tablespoon refined coconut oil,
  melted, or safflower oil, plus more
  for the casserole dish

About 2 tablespoons fine sea salt

1 pound whole wheat or
  brown rice elbow macaroni

2 (10-ounce) packages frozen
  pureed winter squash

2 cups soy or rice milk

4 ounces vegan cheddar cheese,
  shredded

2 ounces vegan Jack cheese,
  shredded

4 ounces (about ½ cup)
  vegan cream cheese

1½ teaspoons powdered mustard

⅛ teaspoon cayenne pepper

¼ cup whole wheat bread crumbs

2 tablespoons vegan Parmesan
  cheese

Preheat oven to 375°F. Oil a 2-quart casserole dish; set aside.

In a 4- to 6-quart stockpot over high heat, combine 3 quarts of water with about 1½ tablespoons of the salt. Bring the water to a boil, add the macaroni, and cook according to the package directions.

Meanwhile, in a 3- to 4-quart saucepan over medium heat, combine the squash and milk, stirring and breaking up the squash with a spoon until the squash is defrosted. Increase the heat to medium-high and bring to a simmer, stirring occasionally. Remove from the heat and whisk in the cheddar, Jack, cream cheese, mustard, cayenne, and the remaining ½ tablespoon of salt.

When the pasta is done, drain it, then return the pasta to the pot. Stir the cheese sauce into the macaroni. Transfer the entire mixture to the prepared baking pan.

In a medium bowl, combine the bread crumbs, Parmesan, and the 1 tablespoon of oil. Sprinkle over the top of the macaroni and cheese. Place the casserole dish on a baking sheet and bake for 20 minutes, then broil for 2 to 3 minutes, or until the top is nicely browned.

> If you don't experience multiple orgasms within the first three bites, you need to see your gyno.

Oven-fried "Chicken" and Cornbread

Serves 6 to 8

Refined coconut oil,
   for the baking sheet

¾ cup whole wheat panko
   (Japanese bread crumbs) or
   whole wheat bread crumbs

⅓ cup vegan chicken bouillon

3 tablespoons cornmeal

½ tablespoon fine sea salt

¾ teaspoon paprika

¼ teaspoon cayenne powder

1 cup soy milk

¾ cup brown rice flour

1½ pounds seitan (in larger blocks
   as opposed to thin slices), broken
   into large hunks

Cornbread (recipe follows)

Preheat oven to 450°F. Grease a large rimmed baking sheet with coconut oil; set aside.

In a shallow bowl, combine the panko, bouillon, corn meal, salt, paprika, and cayenne. Place the soy milk in a second bowl and the rice flour in a third. One at a time, dip the seitan pieces in the soy milk, the rice flour, the soy milk again, and then the panko mixture, pressing to thoroughly coat. Arrange the coated seitan on the prepared baking sheet and bake for 10 minutes. Turn the pieces over and cook another 10 minutes, or until slightly browned and heated throughout. Serve hot with cornbread.

CORNBREAD

Serves 6 to 8

1 tablespoon refined coconut oil,
  melted, or safflower oil, plus more
  for the baking pan

1½ cups yellow cornmeal

1¼ cups whole wheat pastry flour

¾ cup evaporated cane sugar

2 teaspoons baking powder

½ teaspoon fine sea salt

1½ cups soy milk

½ cup silken tofu

Preheat oven to 425°F. Oil a 13 x 9-inch baking pan; set aside.

In a large bowl, combine the cornmeal, flour, sugar, baking powder, and salt. In a blender, combine the milk, tofu, and the 1 tablespoon of the oil, pureeing until smooth. Add the milk mixture to the cornmeal mixture, stirring just until combined. Pour the batter into the prepared baking pan.

Bake the cornbread until golden brown—about 20 minutes. (It'll also begin to pull away from the edges of the pan and spring back when lightly pressed in the center.) Transfer to a cooling rack for 10 minutes, then remove the cornbread from the pan and return to rack to cool completely.

The cornbread can be made in advance and kept at room temperature overnight or in the freezer for up to 1 month.

Cha Cha Chile

Serves 6 to 8

2 cups dry red kidney beans

1 tablespoon refined coconut oil

2 onions, cut into ¼-inch dice

2 cloves garlic, minced

¼ cup chili powder

½ tablespoon fine sea salt

1 teaspoon pepper

1 teaspoon dried oregano

½ teaspoon dried sage

½ teaspoon ground cumin

Pinch cayenne pepper

1 (14½-ounce) can chopped
   tomatoes

½ cup medium-grain brown rice

1 red, green, or yellow bell pepper,
   cut into ¼-inch dice

1 carrot, shredded

Chopped red onion,
   for serving (optional)

Shredded vegan cheddar cheese,
   for serving (optional)

Vegan sour cream, for serving (optional)

In a 4- to 6-quart stockpot, combine the beans and enough cold water to cover by 2 inches. Cover and refrigerate for at least 8 hours or overnight. (Alternately, bring to a boil over high heat, cover, remove from heat, and let sit for 1 hour.)

Drain the beans, return them to the stockpot, and cover with water by 1 inch. Place the pot over high heat, bring to a boil, and reduce to a simmer.

Meanwhile, in an 8- to 10-inch skillet over medium, heat the oil. Add the onions and cook, stirring occasionally, for 4 minutes. Add the garlic, chili powder, salt, pepper, oregano, sage, cumin, and cayenne and cook for 1 minute. Add the onion mixture to the beans, along with the tomatoes and rice. Cook for 30 minutes.

Add the bell pepper and cook for 15 minutes. Add the carrot and cook about 5 minutes, until the beans and rice are tender.

Serve with red onions, shredded cheese, and sour cream, if desired.

Potatoes au Gratin

We thank you Lord, for potatoes. Please forgive our fellow bitches who forsake them. They know not what they do.

Serves 8 to 10

4 medium russet potatoes
  (about 3 pounds), sliced very thin
1 teaspoon fine sea salt
½ teaspoon pepper
4 ounces vegan cheddar cheese,
  shredded
2½ to 3 cups soy creamer
2 tablespoons arrowroot or
  7 teaspoons cornstarch
1½ cups cornflake cereal

Preheat oven to 375°F.

In a 2-quart casserole dish, evenly layer half of the potatoes in a scallop pattern. (You may have to make a couple of layers.) Sprinkle the potatoes with half of the salt, half of the pepper, and half of the cheese. Add the remaining potatoes, evenly layering them in a scallop pattern.

Combine 2½ cups of the creamer with the arrowroot or cornstarch, whisking to dissolve the arrowroot. Pour the mixture over the potatoes. Use a spatula to press the potatoes down into the cream; they should be just barely submerged. If not, add more cream. Sprinkle with the remaining salt, the remaining pepper, and the remaining cheese. Cover and bake for 45 minutes.

Meanwhile, crush the cornflakes, by hand or by pulsing in a food processor, to very coarse crumbs.

Remove the casserole from the oven and use a spatula to moisten the top layer of potatoes by pressing them into the cream. Sprinkle on the cornflakes and bake, uncovered, another 30 to 45 minutes, until the liquid has become a thick sauce, the potatoes are tender, and the cornflakes are browned. Serve warm.

Shepherd's Pie

Serves 6 to 8

1 tablespoon refined coconut oil

2 shallots, thinly sliced

2 cloves garlic, minced

1 teaspoon herbes de Provence
(see page 62)

1 teaspoon fine sea salt

1½ cups lentils

About 3 cups low-sodium
vegetable stock

2 tomatoes, cut into ½-inch dice

1 bunch (about ½ pound) chard,
leafy parts only, cut into ½-inch
strips

6 cups Mashed Potatoes
(see page 119)

Preheat oven to 350°F.

Heat the oil in a 4- to 6-quart stockpot over medium. Add the shallots and cook, stirring occasionally, for 1 minute. Add the garlic, herbes de Provence, and ½ teaspoon of the salt and cook, stirring occasionally, for 1 minute, or until the shallots are browned. Add the lentils and 2½ cups of the vegetable stock, increase the heat to high, and bring to a boil. Reduce to a simmer, cover, and cook until the lentils are tender and the stock is absorbed, 35 to 40 minutes. Stir in the tomatoes and transfer the lentil mixture to a 2-quart casserole dish, spreading it evenly.

Add the remaining ½ cup of stock to the pot and return it to high heat. When the stock comes to a boil, add the chard and the remaining ½ teaspoon of salt. Cook, stirring occasionally, until the chard is tender and the liquid has been absorbed, about 4 minutes. (If the pan gets dry before the chard is cooked, add more stock, 2 tablespoons at a time.) Add the chard to the casserole dish, spreading it evenly. Top with the mashed potatoes, spreading them evenly.

Place the casserole dish on a rimmed baking sheet and bake until thoroughly heated through and the potatoes are slightly browned, about 30 minutes. Serve warm.

If you're feeling fancy, instead of a 2-quart casserole dish, you can serve this in eight 1-cup ramekins. Divide the ingredients among them and check them after only 20 minutes in the oven.

Cheezy Casserole

Serves 6 to 8

Refined coconut oil,
   for the casserole dish

1½ cups short grain brown rice

3 quarts plus 3 cups water

About 4¾ teaspoons fine sea salt

8 ounces (or four to six) red
   potatoes, cut into ¾-inch cubes

2 carrots, cut on a diagonal
   into ¼-inch slices

½ red onion, cut into ¾-inch dice

4 ounces sugar snap peas, cut
   crosswise in half

1 broccoli crown, cut into bite-sized
   florets (about 2½ cups)

14 to 16 ounces firm, extra firm, or
   baked tofu, cut into ½-inch cubes

2¾ cups Cheezy Sauce
   (see page 150)

¼ cup coarsely chopped
   Italian parsley

⅓ cup sliced almonds

Tamari or soy sauce,
   for serving (optional)

Preheat oven to 375°F. Grease a 2-quart casserole dish. Line a large bowl with one or two paper towels.

In a 2-quart saucepan over high heat, combine the rice, 3 cups of the water, and ¼ teaspoon of the salt. Bring to a boil, reduce the heat to a simmer, cover, and cook until the water is absorbed and the rice is tender, about 45 minutes. Remove from the heat and let the rice stand, covered, at least 10 minutes.

Meanwhile, in a 4- to 6-quart stockpot over high heat, combine the remaining 3 quarts of water with about 1½ tablespoons salt. Bring the water to a boil. Add the potatoes and cook until they are soft but still holding their shape, about 5 minutes. Use a slotted spoon or hand-held strainer to remove the potatoes to the prepared bowl. Then remove the paper towels. Add the carrots and onion to the stockpot and cook until tender, about 2 minutes. Use the same slotted spoon to remove the carrots and onions, adding them to the bowl. Add the snap peas and broccoli to the stockpot and cook until tender, about 1 minute. Remove the snap peas and broccoli, adding them to the bowl.

Add the cooked rice, tofu, Cheezy Sauce, and parsley to the vegetables, tossing until combined. Transfer the mixture to the prepared casserole dish. Place the casserole on a rimmed baking sheet and bake for 30 minutes. Sprinkle almonds on top and bake for 15 minutes, or until the almonds are toasted and the tip of a knife inserted into the center of the casserole comes out piping hot. If using, pass the tamari or soy sauce at the table.

"Meatloaf"
with Mashed Potatoes and Gravy

Serves 6

1 tablespoon refined coconut oil,
  plus more for the pan

1 carrot, cut into ¼-inch dice

1 celery stalk, cut into ¼-inch dice

1 onion, cut into ¼-inch dice

3 ounces cremini, shiitake, or
  portobello mushrooms, cut into
  ¼-inch dice (about 2 cups)

2 cloves garlic, minced

2 teaspoons fine sea salt

1 teaspoon pepper

2 slices vegan whole wheat bread

1 cup toasted walnuts

2 (14-ounce) packages Gimme
  Lean vegan ground beef

½ cup rolled oats

½ cup ketchup

2 tablespoons chopped
  fresh Italian parsley

6 cups Mashed Potatoes
  (recipe follows)

2½ cups Brown Gravy (see page 149)

Preheat oven to 375°F. Oil a 10 x 4 x 3 inch loaf pan.

In an 8- to 10-inch skillet over medium heat, melt the oil. Add the carrot and celery and cook, stirring occasionally, for 2 minutes. Add the onion and cook, stirring occasionally, for 3 minutes. Add the mushrooms, garlic, salt, and pepper and cook, stirring occasionally, until the vegetables are crisp-tender and any liquid the mushrooms have released is cooked off, about 2 minutes. Remove from heat and allow to cool slightly.

Meanwhile, in a food processor, combine the bread and walnuts, pulsing to form a coarse meal. Transfer the mixture to a large bowl and add the beef, oats, ketchup, parsley, and the vegetable mixture. Use your hands to mix well. Transfer the loaf mixture to the prepared pan, spread it into an even layer, and bake for 45 minutes, until the tip of a knife inserted into the center comes out piping hot.

Let the loaf sit 5 minutes before turning it out onto a serving plate. Cut into slices and serve with Mashed Potatoes and Brown Gravy. If you're not drooling, check your pulse.

....

MASHED POTATOES

Makes 6 cups, serves 6 to 8

2 quarts water

About 3½ teaspoons fine sea salt

3 large russet potatoes (about 2¼ pounds), cut into 1½-inch cubes

1 cup soy or rice milk

3 tablespoons vegan butter

½ teaspoon pepper

In a 4- to 6-quart stockpot, combine the water and about 1 tablespoon of the salt. Add the potatoes and place the pot over high heat. Bring to a boil, reduce to a simmer, and cook until the potatoes are very tender, 15 to 20 minutes.

Drain the potatoes and return them to the pot. Add the milk, the remaining ½ teaspoon salt, the butter, and pepper. Then mash, bitches, mash!

Sloppy Joes

Serves 4 to 6

2 tablespoons refined coconut oil

1 green bell pepper, cut into
¼-inch dice

1 stalk celery, halved lengthwise
and cut into ¼-inch slices

2 large onions, cut into ¼-inch dice

4 ounces thinly sliced white or
cremini (brown) mushrooms
(about 2 cups)

1 teaspoon chili powder

½ teaspoon fine sea salt

¼ teaspoon pepper

2 cups water

1 (15-ounce) can tomato sauce

¼ cup Bragg's Liquid Aminos (or 8
teaspoons tamari or soy sauce)

¼ cup ketchup

1½ cups textured soy protein

4 to 6 vegan whole wheat
hamburger buns

2 to 3 tablespoons vegan Parmesan
cheese, for serving (optional)

Heat the coconut oil in a 10- to 12-inch skillet over medium high. Add the bell pepper and celery and cook, stirring occasionally, for 2 minutes. Add the onion and cook, stirring occasionally, for 4 minutes. Add the mushroom, chili powder, salt, and pepper and cook, stirring occasionally, for 2 minutes. Stir in the water, tomato sauce, Bragg's Liquid Aminos or tamari or soy sauce, and ketchup. Stir in the textured soy protein, increase the heat to high, and bring to a boil. Reduce to a simmer and cook, stirring occasionally, for 20 minutes.

Meanwhile, split and toast the buns.

To serve, place two bun halves on each plate, open faced. Top the buns with the Sloppy Joe mixture, dividing evenly. Sprinkle with Parmesan cheese, if using, and serve.

Serve with potato salad (see page 66) and dill pickle chips.

Potato Skins with all the Fixin's

Serves 4 to 6 as an appetizer

3 medium russet potatoes, scrubbed and patted dry

Refined coconut oil, for the potatoes and the baking sheet

6 slices vegan bacon, cooked according to package directions

4 ounces shredded vegan cheddar cheese (about 1¼ cups)

4 ounces shredded vegan Jack cheese (about 1¼ cups)

1 tablespoon chopped fresh parsley

½ teaspoon fine sea salt

¼ teaspoon pepper

3 scallions, thinly sliced

¾ cup vegan sour cream

Preheat oven to 425°F.

Rub the potatoes with oil and place them on a large rimmed baking sheet. Bake until the potatoes are tender, about 1 hour. Set the potatoes aside until they're cool enough to handle, but keep the oven on.

Meanwhile, chop the bacon. In a medium bowl, combine the bacon, cheddar cheese, Jack cheese, and parsley; set aside.

Cut each potato lengthwise into quarters. Scoop out the insides, leaving a ¼-inch layer of potato on the skins (save the insides for another use). Oil the baking sheet. Place the skins, skin side down and one inch apart, on the sheet. Sprinkle with the salt, pepper, and the cheese mixture, dividing them evenly. Bake until the skins are crisp and the cheese is melted, about 15 minutes.

Transfer the skins to plates or a platter. Sprinkle with the scallions and dollop with sour cream, dividing evenly.

Skinny Bitch
STAPLE MEALS

These hearty, wholesome, satisfying meals
are the staples to get you through day-to-day life.

Steamed Veggies and Tofu with Brown Rice

Double-dip Fondue

Roasted Sausage, Peppers, Onions,
and Garlic over Soft Polenta

Big-ass Veggie Burrito

Smoked Tofu Stir-Fry

Summer Garden Pasta

Waldorf Wheat Berry Salad

French Lentil Salad

Tamari-roasted Root Vegetables with Cashew Millet

Balsamic Portobello Mushrooms
over Grilled Vegetable Couscous

Spaghetti Squash with Spicy Braised
Greens, Raisins, and Pine Nuts

Hummus, Tempeh, and Cucumber Wrap

Green Goddess Pasta

Chicken Square Meal with White Beans,
Quinoa Pilaf, and Asparagus

Steamed Veggies and Tofu with Brown Rice

Serves 4 to 6

1½ cups medium grain brown rice

3½ cups water, plus more for steaming

¼ teaspoon fine sea salt

½ cup tahini (sesame seed paste)

¼ cup sesame oil

6 tablespoons Bragg's Liquid Aminos, plus more for the table (or 4 tablespoons tamari or soy sauce)

2 carrots, cut into ¼-inch slices

¼ head cauliflower, cut into bite-sized florets (about 2 cups)

¼ head red cabbage (about 6 ounces), cut into ¼-inch strips

¼ bunch kale (about 4 ounces or four to six leaves) cut into ½-inch strips

1 broccoli crown, cut into bite-sized florets (about 2½ cups)

7 to 8 ounces firm or extra firm tofu, cut into ¼-inch slices, then cut on a diagonal into triangles

¼ cup raw pine nuts

In a 2-quart saucepan over high heat, combine the rice, 3 cups of the water, and the salt. Bring to a boil, reduce the heat to a simmer, cover, and cook until the water is absorbed and the rice is tender, about 45 minutes. Remove from the heat and let the rice stand, covered, at least 10 minutes.

Meanwhile, in a small bowl, whisk together the tahini, sesame oil, ¼ cup of the Bragg's Liquid Aminos (or 8 teaspoons of tamari or soy sauce), and the remaining ½ cup of water; set aside.

In a pot fitted with a steamer insert, bring 1 inch of water and the remaining 2 tablespoons of Bragg's Liquid Aminos (or 4 teaspoons of the tamari or soy sauce) to a boil. Arrange the carrot and cauliflower in the insert and steam for 3 minutes. Add the cabbage, kale, broccoli, and tofu and steam for 3 minutes, until the vegetables are tender and the tofu is heated through.

To serve, place the rice on plates or a platter and top with the vegetable mixture, tahini sauce, and pine nuts. Pass any remaining sauce and additional Bragg's Liquid Aminos at the table.

Uhhh!!! This dish tastes so simple, pure, and good it makes us mad!

Double-dip Fondue

Serves 6

2 cups bite-sized broccoli
   florets, blanched

2 cups bite-sized cauliflower
   florets, blanched

2 red bell peppers,
   cut into 1-inch dice

12 bite-sized potatoes, cooked

1½ cups dry white wine

1 tablespoon coarse nutritional yeast

1 clove garlic, pressed or finely
   minced

2 teaspoons Bragg's Liquid
   Aminos, (or 1¼ teaspoons tamari
   or soy sauce)

6 teaspoons arrowroot or
   7 teaspoons cornstarch

6 teaspoons water, divided

1 pound vegan Jack cheese, shredded

2½ cups low-sodium vegetable stock

2 (14- to 16-ounce packages)
   firm or extra firm tofu, pressed
   and cut into ¾-inch cubes

To blanch vegetables: Bring a pot of well-salted water (about ½ tablespoon fine sea salt per quart of water) to a boil. Add the vegetables and cook until crisp-tender, 1 to 3 minutes depending on the vegetable and the size (blanch different vegetables separately since cooking times may vary). Remove with a slotted spoon (if blanching other vegetables) or drain.

To make the cheese fondue: In a 3- to 4-quart saucepan over medium heat, combine the wine, nutritional yeast, garlic, and ½ teaspoon of the Bragg's Liquid Aminos (or ¼ teaspoon tamari or soy sauce), and bring to a simmer.

Meanwhile, in a small bowl, whisk together 4 teaspoons of the arrowroot, (or 4½ teaspoons of the cornstarch) and 4 teaspoons of the water.

About a cup at a time, add the cheese to the saucepan, whisking until all the cheese is incorporated and the mixture is smooth. Whisk in the arrowroot mixture. Bring to a simmer and cook, whisking occasionally, until thickened, 5 to 8 minutes. Transfer to a fondue pot set over a flame.

To make the broth fondue: In a 3- to 4-quart saucepan over medium high heat, combine the stock and the remaining 1½ teaspoons Bragg's Liquid Aminos (or 1 teaspoon tamari or soy sauce), and bring to a simmer.

Meanwhile, in a small bowl, whisk together the remaining 2 teaspoons arrowroot (or 2½ teaspoons of the cornstarch) and the remaining 2 teaspoons water. Whisk the arrowroot mixture into the stock mixture, stirring until slightly thickened. Transfer to a fondue pot set over a flame.

Arrange the broccoli, cauliflower, bell pepper, potatoes, and tofu on plates or a platter and serve.

FYI: The broth is more like a flavorful liquid to warm the veggies and tofu in, while the cheese is more of a dipping thing.

Other things that'd be good to dip: cubed apples, pears, bread, etc.

Roasted Sausage, Peppers, Onions, and Garlic over Soft Polenta

Serves 4

12 cloves garlic

4 red, yellow, or green bell peppers, or a combination, cut into ¾-inch strips

2 onions, quartered and cut into ¾-inch strips

2 tablespoons refined coconut oil, melted, or safflower oil

1 teaspoon fine sea salt

¼ teaspoon pepper

4 (12 to 16 ounces total) vegan Italian sausages, cut diagonally into ¾-inch slices

4 to 4½ cups low-sodium vegetable stock

1 cup polenta

⅔ cup vegan Parmesan cheese

Aged balsamic vinegar or extra virgin olive oil, for drizzling (optional)

Preheat oven to 425°F.

In a large bowl, combine the garlic, bell peppers, onions, oil, ½ teaspoon of the salt, and the pepper, tossing to coat. Transfer the mixture to a rimmed baking sheet and cook for 20 minutes, until the garlic and vegetables are tender.

Stir in the sausages and cook until the vegetables and sausages start to brown, 15 to 20 minutes.

Meanwhile, in a 2- to 3-quart saucepan over medium-high heat, combine 4 cups of the stock and the remaining ½ teaspoon of salt and bring to a boil. Add the polenta in a thin stream, stirring constantly. Return to a boil, reduce to a simmer, cover, and cook until the polenta is tender, 8 to 10 minutes. If the polenta seems too thick, add more stock, ¼ cup at a time. Remove the saucepan from the heat and stir in ⅓ cup of the Parmesan.

To serve, transfer the polenta to 4 serving bowls and top with the sausage and vegetable mixture, dividing evenly. Pass the remaining ⅓ cup of Parmesan and balsamic vinegar or olive oil, if using, at the table.

Big-Ass Veggie Burrito

Makes 4

1 cup brown rice

2 cups water

½ teaspoon plus a pinch fine sea salt

1 (15-ounce) can black beans

1 tablespoon refined coconut oil

1 yellow squash, cut into
   ½-inch cubes

1 green bell pepper, cut into
   ½-inch dice

1 mild green chile, such as pasilla or
   Anaheim, cut into ½-inch dice

½ red onion, cut into ½-inch dice

1 zucchini, quartered lengthwise
   and cut into ½-inch slices

4 cloves garlic, minced

1 teaspoon chili powder

1 teaspoon ground coriander

1 teaspoon ground cumin

2 tomatoes, cut into ½-inch cubes

2 tablespoons lime juice

4 (12- to 14-inch) whole wheat
   tortillas, heated

1 pound vegan cheddar or Jack
   cheese, shredded

½ cup coarsely chopped fresh
   cilantro

2 scallions, thinly sliced

In a 1- to 2-quart saucepan over high heat, combine the rice, water, and a pinch of the salt. Bring to a boil, reduce the heat to a simmer, cover, and cook until the water is absorbed and the rice is tender, about 45 minutes. Remove from the heat and let the rice stand, covered, at least 10 minutes.

Meanwhile, place the beans and their liquid in a 1-quart saucepan over medium heat. Bring to a simmer, reduce the heat to low, and cook until the beans are heated through, about 3 minutes. Cover and set aside.

Heat the coconut oil in a 10- to 12-inch skillet over medium high. Add the squash and cook, stirring occasionally, for 1 minute. Add the bell pepper and chile and cook, stirring occasionally for 1 minute. Add the onion and cook, stirring occasionally, for 2 minutes. Add the zucchini, garlic, chili powder, coriander, cumin, and the remaining ½ teaspoon of salt and cook, stirring occasionally, for 4 minutes, or until all the vegetables are crisp tender. Stir in the tomatoes. Reduce the heat to low, cover, and cook for 4 minutes, until the vegetables are very soft. Stir in the lime juice.

To serve, lay a tortilla on a work surface and top with ¼ of the rice, arranging it in a column down the middle of the tortilla, 2 inches from either edge. Top with ¼ of the beans, ¼ of the vegetable mixture, ¼ of the cheese, ¼ of the cilantro, and ¼ of the scallions. Fold one side of the tortilla up and over the fillings, fold in the edges, and continue rolling the tortilla to the other side, making a tight bundle. Transfer the burrito to a plate, seam down. Repeat with remaining tortillas.

Beans, onions, garlic. You may want to stay in for the night after this one.

Smoked Tofu Stir-fry

Serves 3 to 4

1 cup brown basmati rice

1¾ cups water

Pinch fine sea salt

⅔ cup vegetable stock

¼ cup mirin (see note on page 89)

2 tablespoons tamari or soy sauce,
plus more for the table

1 tablespoon arrowroot
or 3½ teaspoons cornstarch

1 tablespoon refined coconut oil

½ white or yellow onion, halved and
cut into ¼-inch slices

2 heads baby bok choy (about 12
ounces), halved lengthwise then
cut crosswise into ½-inch slices

2 cloves garlic, thinly sliced

1 tablespoon minced ginger

1 portobello mushroom, halved and
cut into ¼-inch slices

8 shiitake mushrooms, stemmed
and thinly sliced

8 white or cremini (brown)
mushrooms, thinly sliced

1 (6- to 8-ounce package) smoked
tofu, cut into bite-sized ¼-inch slices

3 scallions, cut into 2-inch lengths,
white parts halved lengthwise

In a 1- to 2-quart saucepan over high heat, combine the rice, water, and salt. Bring to a boil, reduce the heat to a simmer, cover, and cook until the water is absorbed and the rice is tender, about 30 minutes. Remove from the heat and let the rice stand, covered, at least 10 minutes.

Meanwhile, in a small bowl, whisk together the stock, mirin, tamari or soy sauce, and arrowroot or cornstarch; set aside.

Heat the coconut oil in a 12- to 14-inch wok or skillet over high. Add the onion and stir-fry for 1 minute. Add the bok choy, garlic, and ginger and stir-fry for 1 minute. Add the portobello and stir fry for 1 minute. Add the remaining mushrooms and stir-fry for 3 minutes, or until all the mushrooms are tender. Stir in the stock mixture and the tofu and stir-fry until the tofu is heated through and the sauce has thickened, 1 to 2 minutes. Stir in the scallions.

To serve, arrange the rice on plates or a platter and top with the mushroom mixture. Pass additional tamari or soy sauce at the table.

Summer Garden Pasta

Serves 4

3 quarts water

About 5 teaspoons fine sea salt

8 ounces whole wheat or brown rice linguini or fettuccini

¼ cup refined coconut oil

6 shallots, thinly sliced

1 zucchini, halved lengthwise and thinly sliced

1 yellow squash, halved lengthwise and thinly sliced

4 cloves garlic, thinly sliced

¼ teaspoon pepper

2 pounds tomatoes — red, yellow, or a combination — seeded and cut into coarse ¼-inch dice (about three cups)

½ cup thinly sliced fresh basil leaves

2 tablespoons chopped fresh oregano

¼ cup extra virgin olive oil

1 to 2 tablespoons vegan Parmesan (optional)

In a 4- to 6-quart stockpot over high heat, combine the water with about 1½ tablespoons of the salt. Bring the water to a boil, add the pasta, and cook according to the package directions.

Meanwhile, heat the coconut oil in a 10- to 12-inch skillet over medium high heat. Add the shallots and cook, stirring occasionally, for 3 minutes. Add the zucchini, squash, garlic, pepper, and the remaining ½ teaspoon salt and cook, stirring occasionally, until the vegetables are tender, about 2 minutes. Reduce the heat to medium and add the tomatoes, basil, and oregano, stirring until the tomatoes are heated through, about 2 minutes.

When the pasta is done, drain it. Transfer the pasta to plates or a platter and top with the tomato mixture. Drizzle with olive oil, sprinkle with Parmesan, if using, and serve.

Waldorf Wheat Berry Salad

Serves 6 to 8

1 cup hard wheat berries (see note)

3 cups water, plus more for soaking

⅓ cup safflower oil

¼ cup apple juice

2 tablespoons rice vinegar

2 tablespoons agave nectar

¾ teaspoon fine sea salt

½ teaspoon pepper

2 celery stalks, thinly sliced

2 scallions, thinly sliced

1 sweet-tart apple, such as Fuji,
   Jonathan, or McIntosh,
   cut into ½-inch cubes

½ small red onion,
   cut into ¼-inch dice

½ cup dried cranberries

½ cup chopped pecans

½ cup chopped fresh Italian parsley

HARD WHEAT BERRIES
are available in the bulk section
of natural food stores and
many supermarkets.

In a 2- to 3-quart saucepan, combine the wheat berries and enough water to cover by 2 inches and soak, refrigerated, for 6 hours or overnight. (If you don't have time for the overnight drama, use ½ cup more water and cook for thirty minutes more, or until tender.)

Drain the wheat berries, return them to the pot, and add the 3 cups of water. Bring to a boil over high heat, reduce the heat to a simmer, cover, and cook for 50 to 60 minutes, until the berries are tender.

Meanwhile, in a small bowl, whisk together the safflower oil, apple juice, rice vinegar, agave, salt, and pepper. Once the berries are cooked, drain any water left in the pot and transfer the berries to a large bowl. Toss with about half the dressing and set aside to cool to room temperature.

Once the berries are cool, stir in the ingredients and remaining dressing, tossing gently. Serve cold.

French Lentil Salad

Serves 6 to 8

1 cup French green lentils (see note)

2 cups water

6 tablespoons extra virgin olive oil

2 tablespoons white wine vinegar
  or champagne vinegar

½ tablespoon fresh chopped or
  ½ teaspoon dry tarragon

1 teaspoon Dijon mustard

1 teaspoon fine sea salt

½ teaspoon pepper

2 tomatoes, cut into ½-inch dice

2 large Belgian endive (about 8
  ounces), halved lengthwise and
  cut into ½-inch slices

1 green bell pepper,
  cut into ½-inch dice

1 yellow bell pepper, cut into
  ½-inch dice

½ cup chopped fresh Italian parsley

In a 1- to 2-quart saucepan over high, combine the lentils and water and bring to a boil. Reduce the heat to a simmer, cover, and cook 35 to 45 minutes, until the lentils are al dente, tender but not mushy.

Meanwhile, in a small bowl, whisk together the olive oil, vinegar, tarragon, mustard, salt, and pepper.

Once the lentils are cooked, drain any water left in the pot and transfer the lentils to a large bowl. Toss with about half the dressing and set aside to cool to room temperature.

Once the lentils are cool, stir in the tomatoes, endive, bell peppers, and parsley. Add the remaining dressing, tossing gently. Serve cold or at room temperature.

Don't get all psycho if you can't find French green lentils. This can be made with brown, pink, or regular green lentils, as well.

Tamari-roasted Root Vegetables with Cashew Millet

Serves 6

4 beets (about 24 ounces), trimmed, peeled, and cut into ¾-inch cubes

4 rutabagas (about 24 ounces), trimmed, peeled, and cut into ¾-inch cubes

4 turnips (about 24 ounces), trimmed, peeled, and cut into ¾-inch cubes

3 tablespoons tamari, plus more for the table

1 tablespoon safflower oil

3¾ cups low-sodium vegetable stock

1½ cups hulled millet

¼ teaspoon fine sea salt

½ cup chopped cashews

Preheat oven to 375°F.

In a large bowl, combine the beets, rutabagas, turnips, tamari, and safflower oil. Spread the mixture onto two large rimmed baking sheets and bake for 30 minutes. One pan at a time, remove the pans from the oven, toss the vegetables, and spread them back out. Cook for another 30 minutes, or until the vegetables are tender and nicely caramelized.

Meanwhile, in a 3- to 4-quart saucepan over high heat, combine the stock, millet, and salt. Bring to a boil, reduce the heat to a simmer, cover, and cook for 15 minutes, or until the millet is tender. Remove from the heat, fluff with a fork, cover, and set aside until the vegetables are done.

To serve, transfer the millet to plates or a platter, top with the vegetables, and sprinkle with cashews. Pass additional tamari at the table.

Balsamic Portobello Mushrooms over Grilled Vegetable Couscous

Serves 4

¾ cup coconut oil, melted,
   or safflower oil

½ cup balsamic vinegar

2 tablespoons maple syrup

2 tablespoons chopped
   fresh rosemary

½ teaspoon freshly ground
   black pepper

2¼ teaspoons fine sea salt

1 small red onion

4 portobello mushrooms

1 medium zucchini, cut lengthwise
   into ½-inch slices

1 yellow squash, cut lengthwise
   into ½-inch slices

1¼ cups water

1 cup couscous

In a medium bowl, whisk together the oil, balsamic vinegar, maple syrup, rosemary, pepper, and ½ tablespoon of the salt; set aside.

Trim the stem end off of onion and peel. Cut the onion into 8 wedges, each with a bit of the root end holding it together. Place the onion, portobellos, zucchini, and squash in a large, resealable bag and add the balsamic mixture. Press the air out of the bag, seal, and set aside for 2 to 4 hours, turning occasionally.

Prepare an outdoor or stovetop grill to medium heat (it's at the right temperature when you can hold your hand grate-level for 4 seconds).

Remove the vegetables from the bag and reserve 2 tablespoons of the marinade (save the rest for another use). Grill the vegetables for 8 to 10 minutes, turning once, until well-marked and tender.

(If you don't have a grill, use two to three skillets with a little oil in the bottom over medium-high heat. Just be sure not to crowd the veggies in there or they'll steam instead of sear.

Meanwhile, in a 2- to 3-quart saucepan over medium heat, bring the water and the remaining ¾ teaspoon of salt to a boil. Stir in the couscous, cover, remove from the heat, and let stand for 5 minutes.

Once the vegetables have cooked, coarsely chop the onion, zucchini, and squash. Stir the chopped vegetables into the couscous, along with the reserved marinade. Cut the portobellos into thick slices.

Arrange the couscous on plates or a platter, top with the portobellos and any accumulated juices, and serve.

Spaghetti Squash with Spicy Braised Greens, Raisins, and Pine Nuts

Serves 4

½ of a 4-pound spaghetti squash, with the seeds scraped out (see note)

Water for the baking pan

2 tablespoons refined coconut oil

2 cloves garlic, minced

1 to 2 canned chipotle chiles in adobo sauce, seeded and minced

1½ bunches (about 12 ounces) kale, chard, mustard greens, collard greens, or a combination, cut into ½-inch strips

1 to 1½ cups low-sodium vegetable stock

¾ teaspoon fine sea salt

⅓ cup raisins

¼ cup pine nuts

2 tablespoons extra virgin olive oil

Preheat oven to 375°F.

Place the squash flesh down in a 13 x 9-inch baking pan. Add ¼ inch of water and bake until the squash is easily pierced with a fork, 50 to 60 minutes.

Meanwhile, heat the coconut oil in a 4- to 6-quart stockpot over medium. Add the garlic and chipotle and cook for 1 minute. Add the greens, handfuls at a time, stirring until they're all in the pot. Add 1 cup of the stock, ½ teaspoon of the salt, and the raisins. Increase the heat to high and bring to a boil. Reduce the heat to a simmer, cover, and cook until the greens are tender, about 10 minutes, or 15 to 20 minutes for collard greens. (If the pan gets dry before the chard is cooked, add more stock, 2 tablespoons at a time.) Stir in 3 tablespoons of the pine nuts.

When the squash is done, use a fork to separate the strands into a large bowl.

Add the olive oil and the remaining ¼ teaspoon of salt and toss gently.

Transfer the "spaghetti" to plates or a platter, top with the greens mixture, garnish with the remaining 1 tablespoon of pine nuts, and serve.

We're not dumb broads. We know that "½ of a 4-pound squash" means you could just buy a 2-pound squash. But a larger squash merits longer, thicker strands of spaghetti than a whole small squash. So do what you're told— just save the other half for another use

Hummus, Tempeh, and Cucumber Wrap

Makes 4

1 tablespoon refined coconut oil

½ teaspoon garlic powder

¼ teaspoon ground coriander

2 tablespoons tamari or soy sauce

1 (8-ounce) package tempeh, cut lengthwise into ¼-inch strips

4 (9- to 10-inch) whole wheat tortillas

1 cup hummus

1 cucumber, peeled and cut diagonally into ¼-inch slices

1 romaine heart, cut into ½-inch strips

¼ cup bottled vinaigrette dressing, whatever kind you like

Heat the coconut oil in a 10- to 12-inch skillet over medium heat. Stir in the garlic powder, coriander, and tamari or soy sauce. Add the tempeh and cook 1½ to 2 minutes per side, until browned.

To serve, lay a tortilla on a work surface and spread it with ¼ of the hummus. Arrange ¼ of the tempeh in a column down the middle of the tortilla, leaving a 2-inch border on one edge. Top with ¼ of the cucumber, ¼ of the romaine, and ¼ of the dressing. Fold one side of the tortilla up and over the fillings, fold in the edge with the border, and continue rolling the tortilla to the other side, making a tight bundle. Transfer the wrap to a plate or a platter, seam down. Repeat with the remaining tortillas.

Green Goddess Pasta

Serves 4

4 cloves garlic, minced

3 tablespoons refined coconut oil

6 tablespoons vegan butter

3 quarts water

About 5 teaspoons fine sea salt

8 ounces whole wheat or brown rice
   elbow macaroni

2 zucchini, halved lengthwise and
   cut into ¼-inch slices

1 broccoli crown, cut into bite-sized
   florets (about 2½ cups)

½ bunch (about 4 ounces) kale, cut
   into ½-inch strips

½ teaspoon pepper

¼ cup pine nuts

In a 1-quart saucepan over low heat, combine the garlic and coconut oil and cook, swirling occasionally, until the garlic is fragrant and starting to brown, about 3 minutes. Remove from the heat, add the butter, swirling until it melts, and set aside.

In a 4- to 6-quart stockpot over high heat, combine the water with about 1½ tablespoons salt. Bring the water to a boil, add the macaroni, and cook according to the package directions until about 1 minute shy of being done. Stir in the zucchini, broccoli, and kale. Cook until the vegetables are tender and the pasta is cooked, about 1 minute.

Drain the pasta mixture, reserving ½ cup of the pasta cooking water. Return the mixture to the pot and stir in the garlic butter, pepper, 3 tablespoons of the pine nuts, and the remaining ½ teaspoon of salt. Transfer the pasta to plates or a platter, garnish with remaining 1 tablespoon of pine nuts, and serve.

"Chicken" Square Meal with White Beans, Quinoa Pilaf, and Asparagus

Serves 6

1½ cups dried small white beans

2 cloves garlic, smashed

1 bay leaf

2 tablespoons extra virgin olive oil

1½ teaspoons fine sea salt

½ tablespoon refined coconut oil
  or safflower oil

1 cup quinoa

2 cups low-sodium vegetable stock

1 cup frozen mixed vegetables
  (no need to thaw)

6 vegan chicken cutlets

1 bunch (about 1 pound)
  asparagus, trimmed

1 lemon, cut into wedges,
  for garnish

In a 3-quart saucepan, combine the beans and enough cold water to cover by 1 inch. Cover and refrigerate for at least 8 hours or overnight. (Alternately, bring to a boil over high heat, cover, remove from heat, and let sit for 1 hour.)*

Drain the beans, return them to the saucepan, and cover with water by 1 inch. Add the garlic and bay leaf. Place the pot over high heat, bring to a boil, and reduce to a simmer. Cover and cook until the beans are tender, about 25 minutes. Remove from the heat, drain any water left in the pot, and stir in the olive oil and ¾ teaspoon of the salt.

Meanwhile, in a 2- to 3-quart saucepan over medium-high, melt the coconut oil. Add the quinoa and cook, stirring occasionally, until the quinoa is browned, about 5 minutes. Stir in the stock, the mixed vegetables, and ¼ teaspoon of the salt. Bring to a boil, reduce the heat to a simmer, cover, and cook until the stock is absorbed and the quinoa is tender, about 20 minutes.

While the beans and quinoa are cooking, cook the chicken according to package directions.

When everything is about 10 minutes from being done, in an 8- to 10-inch skillet over high heat, combine ½-inch of water and the remaining ½ teaspoon of salt and bring to a simmer. Add the asparagus and cook, turning occasionally and adjusting the heat to maintain a simmer, until crisp-tender, 3 to 5 minutes, depending on the size of the asparagus.

Transfer the chicken, beans, quinoa, and asparagus to 4 serving plates, dividing evenly. Garnish with lemon wedges and serve.

*For all you bitches in a rush: Instead of dried beans, you can use canned beans. Substitute 2 (15-ounce) cans of white beans. Place the beans and their liquid in 1- to 2-quart saucepan over medium heat. Bring to a simmer, reduce the heat to low, and cook until the beans are heated through, about 5 minutes. Cover and set aside until ready to serve— then, either drain the beans or serve them with a slotted spoon.

Divine Dressings, SAUCES, AND SUBSTITUTES

If you have shitty taste buds from eating poorly all these years, healthy food may not taste so good to you. If that's the case, douse your grub with any one of these gooey delights.

Savory White Cream Sauce

Brown Gravy

Cheezy Sauce

Ranch Dressing

Thousand Island Dressing

Miso-Ginger Dressing

Agave-Dijon Spread

Agave-Dijon Dressing

Vegan Caesar Dressing

Basil Pesto

Sage Pesto

Basic Red Sauce

Super Simple Pizza Sauce

Tofu "Ricotta"

Marinated Tofu "Feta"

Savory White Cream Sauce

Makes about 2 cups

About 2 cups soy or rice milk

¼ cup refined coconut oil

½ onion, finely diced

¼ cup whole wheat pastry flour

½ teaspoon fine sea salt

¼ teaspoon white pepper

⅛ teaspoon ground nutmeg

In a 1-quart saucepan over low heat, heat 2 cups of soy milk until it's barely simmering (small bubbles will appear at the edges of the pan). Cover and set aside.

Heat the oil in a 2- to 3-quart saucepan over medium heat. Add the onion and cook, stirring occasionally, until tender, 4 to 6 minutes. Whisk in the flour and cook, whisking constantly, for 2 minutes. Slowly whisk in the hot milk and bring the mixture to a simmer. Reduce the heat to low and cook, whisking often, until the sauce is thick and no longer tastes of raw flour, 6 to 8 minutes. Remove from the heat and whisk in the salt, pepper, and nutmeg. If not using immediately, transfer the sauce to a bowl, cover with plastic wrap directly on the surface of the sauce, and use within 30 minutes. If the sauce gets too thick while it sits, whisk in a little more warm soy milk.

Brown Gravy

Makes about 2½ cups

¼ cup refined coconut oil

½ cup whole wheat pastry flour

2 to 2¼ cups low-sodium
vegetable stock

4 tablespoons Bragg's Liquid
Aminos (or 8 teaspoons tamari or
soy sauce)

Heat the oil in a 2- to 3-quart saucepan over medium heat. When the oil is almost completely melted, whisk in the flour. Cook, stirring often, until the mixture is browned and smells nutty, about 5 minutes. A little at a time, add 2 cups of the stock, whisking until smooth after each addition. Remove from the heat and whisk in the Bragg's Liquid Aminos (or tamari or soy sauce). Add more stock, if desired, until the gravy reaches the desired consistency. Serve hot, or cool, cover, and refrigerate for 3 or 4 days. Reheat gently, adding a little more stock or water if necessary.

Cheezy Sauce

Makes about 2¾ cups

About 2 cups soy or rice milk

¼ cup refined coconut oil

¼ cup whole wheat pastry flour

8 ounces vegan cheese (cheddar, mozzarella, Jack, whatever you like, or a combination), shredded

½ teaspoon fine sea salt

¼ teaspoon white pepper

In a 1-quart saucepan over low heat, heat 2 cups of soy or rice milk until it's barely simmering (small bubbles will appear at the edges of the pan). Cover and set aside.

Heat the oil in a 2- to 3-quart saucepan over medium heat. Whisk in the flour and cook, whisking constantly, for 2 minutes. Slowly whisk in the hot milk and bring the mixture to a simmer. Reduce the heat to low and cook, whisking often, until the sauce is thick and no longer tastes of raw flour, 6 to 8 minutes. Remove from the heat and whisk in the cheese, salt, and pepper, stirring until the cheese melts (if necessary, return the pot to low heat). If not using immediately, transfer the sauce to a bowl, cover with plastic wrap directly on the surface of the sauce, and use within 30 minutes. If the sauce gets too thick while it sits, whisk in a little more warm soy or rice milk.

Ranch Dressing

Makes about 1¾ cups

1 cup vegan sour cream

½ cup soy milk

¼ cup safflower oil

1 tablespoon agave nectar

1 tablespoon granulated
   garlic powder

2 teaspoons chopped dill

1 teaspoon Dijon mustard

1 teaspoon fine sea salt

½ teaspoon onion powder

½ teaspoon cider vinegar

¼ teaspoon pepper

¼ teaspoon tamari or soy sauce

In a blender or a food processor, combine all ingredients and process until smooth. Set aside in the refrigerator overnight to allow the flavors to bloom. Store refrigerated for up to 1 week.

Thousand Island Dressing

Makes about 1⅓ cups

1 cup vegan mayonnaise

¼ cup ketchup

¼ cup sweet pickle relish

2 tablespoons tomato paste

3 tablespoons lemon juice

½ teaspoon fine sea salt

⅛ teaspoon cayenne

In a small bowl, whisk together all the ingredients. Use immediately, or cover and refrigerate for up to 1 week.

Eat. It. With. A. Spoon.

Miso Ginger Dressing

Makes about 1½ cups

¾ cup canola or safflower oil

¼ cup red miso

¼ cup water

2 tablespoons agave nectar

2 tablespoons rice wine vinegar

2 tablespoons grated fresh ginger

1 teaspoon sesame oil

In a small bowl, whisk together all the ingredients. Use immediately, or cover and refrigerate for up to 1 week.

This one's so good it can perk up even the lamest of salads.

Agave-Dijon Spread

Makes ½ cup

¼ cup agave nectar

¼ cup Dijon mustard

In a small bowl, whisk together the agave and mustard. Use immediately, or cover and refrigerate for up to 2 months.

> This spread can be used on all kinds of sandwiches, burgers, and "chicken."

Agave-Dijon Dressing

Makes about 1½ cups

¼ cup agave nectar

¼ cup Dijon mustard

⅔ cup extra virgin olive oil

¼ cup red wine vinegar or balsamic vinegar

2 cloves garlic, minced

½ teaspoon fine sea salt

½ teaspoon pepper

In a small bowl, whisk together all ingredients. Use immediately, or cover and refrigerate for up to 1 month.

> This would totally kick ass on a spinach salad.

Divine Dressings, Sauces, and Substitutes   153

Caesar Dressing

Makes 1½ cups

4 ounces silken tofu

6 tablespoons lemon juice

3 cloves garlic

2 tablespoons vegan
  Parmesan cheese

½ tablespoon Dijon mustard

2 teaspoons vegan
  Worcestershire sauce

½ teaspoon fine sea salt

½ teaspoon pepper

¼ teaspoon kelp powder (optional, to
  give it an anchovy kind of flavor)

¾ cup extra virgin olive oil

In a food processor, combine the tofu, lemon juice, garlic, cheese, mustard, Worcestershire sauce, salt, pepper, and kelp powder, if using, and process until smooth. With the motor running, slowly drizzle in the olive oil. Use immediately, or cover and refrigerate for up to 1 week.

Basil Pesto

Makes about 1⅓ cups

¼ cup pine nuts

4 cloves garlic

3 cups fresh basil leaves

¼ cup vegan Parmesan cheese

½ teaspoon fine sea salt

⅛ teaspoon pepper

¾ cup extra virgin olive oil,
plus more for storing

In a food processor, combine the pine nuts and garlic and pulse to roughly chop. Add the basil and pulse to chop. Add the cheese, salt, and pepper and process into a paste. With the motor running, slowly pour in the olive oil, processing until the oil is fully combined. Use immediately or transfer to a small container, cover with a thin layer of olive oil, and store in the refrigerator for 3 to 4 weeks.

Sage Pesto

Makes about 1 cup

¼ cup whole almonds

2 cloves garlic

1½ cups fresh sage leaves

¾ cup fresh Italian parsley leaves

3 ounces (about ⅓ cup) soy
cream cheese

½ teaspoon fine sea salt

⅛ teaspoon pepper

⅔ cup extra virgin olive oil, plus
more for storing

In a food processor, combine the almonds and garlic and pulse to roughly chop. Add the sage and parsley and pulse to chop. Add the cream cheese, salt, and pepper and process into a paste. With the motor running, slowly pour in the olive oil, processing until the oil is fully combined. Use immediately or transfer to a small container, cover with a thin layer of olive oil, and store in the refrigerator for 3 to 4 weeks.

Basic Red Sauce

Makes about 7 cups

2 tablespoons refined coconut oil

1 onion, cut into ¼-inch dice

8 to 10 cloves garlic, minced

2 (28-ounce) cans crushed tomatoes

1 (6-ounce) can tomato paste

¼ cup fruity red wine (optional)

2 tablespoons finely
chopped fresh basil

1 tablespoon finely
chopped fresh oregano

½ teaspoon salt

⅛ teaspoon hot sauce, like
Tabasco (optional)

1 tablespoon agave nectar
(optional)

Heat the coconut oil in a 4- to 6-quart stockpot over medium-low heat. Add the onion and cook, stirring occasionally, until tender, 6 to 8 minutes (adjust heat, if necessary, to avoid browning). Add the garlic and cook, stirring occasionally, 1 minute. Stir in the tomatoes and tomato paste, increase the heat to high, and bring to a boil. Remove from the heat and stir in the wine, if using, along with the basil, oregano, salt, and hot sauce (if using). Taste, and if the sauce is too acidic, stir in the agave. Use immediately or cover and refrigerate for up to 1 week or freeze for up to 2 months.

Super Simple Pizza Sauce

Makes about 1¾ cup

1 (14.5-ounce) can diced tomatoes

¼ cup tomato paste

2 cloves garlic

2 teaspoons red wine vinegar

1 teaspoon chopped fresh oregano
   or ½ teaspoon dried oregano

½ teaspoon fine sea salt

⅛ teaspoon pepper

⅛ teaspoon cayenne powder

In a food processor, combine all the ingredients and pulse to puree. Use immediately or cover and refrigerate for up to 1 week or freeze for up to 2 months.

Tofu "Ricotta"

Makes about 2 cups

14 to 16 ounces extra firm tofu,
  crumbled

3 cloves garlic

2 tablespoons extra virgin olive oil

1 tablespoon chopped fresh
  oregano or 1 teaspoon dried
  oregano

¾ teaspoon fine sea salt

In a food processor, combine the tofu, garlic, olive oil, oregano, and salt and pulse to puree. Use immediately or cover and refrigerate for up to 1 week.

This is so similar to the real deal it makes us angry. Why is it so good? Why?

Marinated Tofu "Feta"

Makes about 3 cups

2 tablespoons extra virgin olive oil

1½ tablespoons lemon juice

1 teaspoon dried oregano

1 teaspoon fine sea salt

½ teaspoon crushed red pepper

14 to 16 ounces firm or extra firm
tofu, cut into ½- or ¾-inch cubes

In a medium bowl, whisk together the olive oil, lemon juice, oregano, salt, and red pepper. Add the tofu and toss gently. Let marinate for at least 1 hour, stirring occasionally. Use immediately.

Happy
ENDINGS

If eating dessert is wrong, we don't want to be right.
Give us dessert, or give us death. Life without dessert is
like life without the sun. We never met a dessert we didn't
like. Clearly, we're totally fucking psychotic for dessert.

Chocolate Chip Cookies

Peanut Butter Potato Chip Cookies

Buttery Shortbread Cookies

Bitchtastic Brownies

Hot Fudge Brownie Sundaes

Cheezecake

Vanilla Cake with Frosting

Carrot Cake with Cream Cheese Frosting

Chocolate Suicide Cake

Dream Bars

Rice Pudding

Fresh Fruit Crisp

Chocolate Chip Cookies

Makes about 48

2½ cups whole wheat pastry flour

½ tablespoon baking soda

1 teaspoon fine sea salt

1½ cups evaporated cane sugar

1¼ cups refined coconut oil

¼ cup ice water

1 tablespoon molasses

½ tablespoon pure vanilla extract

1 (10- to 12-ounce) package vegan
   chocolate chips

1 cup chopped walnuts (optional)

> Seriously. Can you stand
> these?

Preheat oven to 375°F. Line baking sheets with parchment.

In a medium bowl, sift together the flour, baking soda, and salt; set aside.

In the bowl of a stand mixer or in a large bowl with a hand mixer, combine the sugar and coconut oil, mixing on medium-high speed until creamy, about 3 minutes. Add the water, molasses, and vanilla, mixing until well combined. With the mixer on low speed, add the flour mixture in 3 to 4 additions, mixing each addition until almost fully incorporated. Add in the chocolate chips and the walnuts, if using, mixing until just combined.

Arrange 2-tablespoon-sized balls of cookie dough 2 inches apart on prepared baking sheets. Bake for 13 to 15 minutes, until the edges are slightly browned and the centers are set. Thoroughly cool on a cooling rack.

Peanut Butter Potato Chip Cookies

Makes about 40

2½ cups whole wheat pastry flour

2 teaspoons baking soda

¾ teaspoon fine sea salt

1½ cups evaporated cane sugar

1 cup refined coconut oil

1 cup all-natural peanut butter,
  chunky or smooth (whichever
  you prefer)

¼ cup ice water

1 tablespoon molasses

1 teaspoon pure vanilla extract

2 cups coarsely crushed potato chips

Preheat oven to 375°F. Line baking sheets with parchment.

In a medium bowl, sift together the flour, baking soda, and salt; set aside.

In the bowl of a stand mixer or in a large bowl with a hand mixer, combine the sugar, coconut oil, and peanut butter, mixing on medium-high speed until creamy, about 3 minutes. Add the water, molasses, and vanilla, mixing until well combined. With the mixer on low speed, add the flour mixture in 3 to 4 additions, mixing each addition until almost fully incorporated. Add the potato chips, mixing until just combined.

Arrange 2-tablespoon-sized balls of cookie dough 2 inches apart on prepared baking sheets. Press to about ¾-inch thick, then use the back of a fork to mark each cookie with a crosshatch pattern, if desired. Bake for 13 to 15 minutes, until the edges are slightly browned and the centers are set. Thoroughly cool on a cooling rack. Then eat enough to make yourself sick.

Buttery Shortbread Cookies

Makes about 36 cookies

1¾ cups whole wheat pastry flour

1 tablespoon coarse nutritional yeast

1 teaspoon fine sea salt

½ cup refined coconut oil, cut into pieces if in large chunks

½ cup powdered evaporated cane sugar

1 teaspoon pure vanilla extract

1 tablespoon orange juice

Preheat oven to 325°F. Line baking sheets with parchment.

In a medium bowl, combine the flour, nutritional yeast, and salt; set aside.

In the bowl of a stand mixer or in a large bowl with a hand mixer, cream the coconut oil, mixing on medium-high speed for about 3 minutes. Add the sugar and beat until light and fluffy, about 2 minutes. Add the vanilla and orange juice, mixing until well combined. With the mixer on low speed, add the flour mixture in 3 to 4 additions, mixing until just combined. Transfer the dough to a work surface, shape it into a ¾-inch disk, cover with plastic wrap, and refrigerate until firm enough to roll out, 5 to 10 minutes.

Transfer the dough to a lightly floured work surface and roll out to ¼-inch thick. Cut into shapes and arrange on prepared baking sheets. Reroll the dough and cut into shapes one or two more times. Bake for 20 minutes, or until the edges are just starting to brown.

Bitchtastic Brownies

Makes 9 or 12

5 ounces unsweetened vegan
  chocolate, chopped

1¼ cups Sucanat
  (or other dry sweetener)

¾ cup silken tofu

6 tablespoons safflower oil, plus
  more for the pan

1 tablespoon pure vanilla extract

⅓ cup whole wheat pastry flour

2 tablespoons unsweetened
  cocoa powder

¼ teaspoon refined sea salt

Preheat oven to 350°F. Oil an 8 x 8 inch baking pan; set aside.

In the top of a double boiler or in a medium metal bowl set over a pot of gently simmering water, melt the chocolate, stirring just until smooth. Transfer the chocolate to a food processor and add the Sucanat, tofu, oil, and vanilla; process until smooth. Add the flour, cocoa powder, and salt, pulsing until just combined. Transfer the batter to the prepared pan, spreading it evenly. Bake for 30 minutes, until a toothpick inserted into the center comes out clean. Thoroughly cool on a cooling rack before cutting into 9 or 12 squares.

> Oh please, who are we kidding? Eat 'em while they're hot and burn your friggin' mouths off.

Hot Fudge Brownie Sundaes

Makes 4

4 ounces semi-sweet vegan
   chocolate, chopped

3 tablespoons vegan cream

4 Bitchtastic Brownies
   (preceding page)

1 pint vegan vanilla ice cream

2 tablespoons chopped toasted
   pecans

4 cherries with stems

In the top of a double boiler or in a medium metal bowl set over a pot of gently simmering water, melt the chocolate and cream, stirring just until smooth; set aside.

Arrange the brownies on plates. Top each with a scoop of ice cream then drizzle with the chocolate sauce (you may not need it all) and sprinkle with pecans, dividing evenly. Finish with a cherry on top, and serve.

Cheezecake

Serves 10 to 12

1½ cups vegan cookie crumbs
(see note on next page)

3 tablespoons refined coconut oil,
melted, or safflower oil

1 cup plus 7 tablespoons raw
(turbinado) evaporated cane
sugar (or other dry sweetener)

2 pounds tofu cream cheese

1 pound silken tofu

3 tablespoons arrowroot or
3 tablespoons plus 2 teaspoons
cornstarch

1 tablespoon pure vanilla extract

Zest and juice of 1 lemon

Fruit Glaze Topping
(optional, recipe follows)

Preheat oven to $325\,^{\circ}$F.

In a medium bowl, combine the cookie crumbs, oil, and 3 tablespoons of the sugar, stirring until the mixture is uniformly moist. Transfer to a 10-inch springform pan and press the mixture evenly into the bottom and 1 to 2 inches up the sides of the pan. Place the pan on a rimmed baking sheet and bake until the crust is lightly browned and dry, 15 to 20 minutes. Thoroughly cool on a cooling rack.

While the crust is cooling, increase the oven temperature to $350\,^{\circ}$F.

In the bowl of a food processor, combine about ¼ of the cream cheese and the tofu; process until smooth. Transfer the mixture to the bowl of a stand mixer or a large bowl with a hand mixer. Add the remaining cream cheese and the remaining 1¼ cups sugar and mix on medium speed until smooth.

In a small bowl, combine the arrow-root or cornstarch, vanilla, and lemon juice. Add this mixture, along with the lemon zest, to the cream cheese mixture, beating just until smooth. Pour the entire mixture into the cooled crust. Place the pan on the rimmed baking sheet and bake for 50 minutes.

When time is up, turn off the heat but leave the cheesecake in the oven until the edges are set and lightly browned but the center is still wobbly, about 60 minutes. Remove from the oven, run a knife around the edge of the crust, and let cool completely.

Cover and chill for at least 4 hours and up to a day before removing the sides of the pan. Just before serving, pour the glaze on top, if using, spreading it evenly.

To make cookie crumbs, start with whatever kind of vegan cookies you like — graham crackers, ginger snaps, chocolate wafers, whatever. Put a couple of handfuls in the food processor and pulse until they're finely ground. Repeat until you have 1½ cups (the number of cookies it takes depends on the size and density of the cookie).

FRUIT GLAZE TOPPING

1 cup all-fruit jam or preserves, whatever flavor you like

1 tablespoon arrowroot or 3½ teaspoons cornstarch dissolved in ⅓ cup water

In a small saucepan over medium heat, whisk together the jam and the arrowroot mixture. Bring to a simmer, whisking until thickened and no longer milky-looking, about 3 minutes. Cool thor-oughly before spreading on cooked, cooled, chilled cheesecake.

Vanilla Cake with Frosting

Serves 10 to 12

1 cup refined coconut oil,
   plus more for pans

4 cups whole wheat pastry flour,
   plus more for cake pans

1 tablespoon baking powder

½ teaspoon baking soda

¾ teaspoon fine sea salt

1⅓ cups rice or soy milk

1 cup silken tofu

⅓ cup safflower oil

1½ tablespoons vanilla extract

2 cups evaporated cane sugar
   (or other dry sweetener)

4 cups Vanilla or Chocolate Frosting
   (recipe follows)

> Try not to eat the entire
> batch of frosting before you
> put it on the cake, pig.

Preheat oven to 350°F. Oil and flour two 9-inch cake pans and line the bottoms with parchment. Oil the parchment and dust the pans lightly with flour.

In a medium bowl, sift together the flour, baking powder, baking soda, and salt; set aside.

In a food processor, combine the milk, tofu, safflower oil, and vanilla; set aside.

In the bowl of a stand mixer or in a large bowl with a hand mixer, combine the coconut oil and sugar, mixing on medium-high speed until fluffy, 3 to 5 minutes. With the mixer on low speed, add the flour mixture in 3 additions, alternating with the tofu mixture, mixing until just combined.

Transfer the batter to the prepared pans and smooth the surfaces. Bake for 30 to 35 minutes, or until the cakes spring back when lightly touched in the center and begin to pull away from the sides of the pan. Cool on racks for 10 minutes. Unmold the cakes and return to racks to thoroughly cool.

Spread each cake with about ¼ of the Vanilla Frosting or Fudgy Chocolate Frosting. Stack the cakes, then use the remaining frosting to coat the sides of the cake and your boobs.

VANILLA FROSTING

Makes about 4 cups

½ cup refined coconut oil

8 to 10 tablespoons soy milk
   or nondairy creamer

2 teaspoons vanilla extract

¼ teaspoon salt

8 cups (about 2 pounds) powdered
   evaporated cane sugar

In the bowl of a stand mixer or in a large bowl with a hand mixer, cream the coconut oil, mixing on medium-high speed for about 3 minutes. Add 8 tablespoons of the milk or creamer, the vanilla, and salt, mixing until well combined. With the mixer on low speed, add the sugar, about ½ cup at a time. If the frosting seems too stiff, add 1 to 2 tablespoons more milk. Increase the speed to high and beat until smooth and fluffy, 1 to 2 minutes.

FUDGY CHOCOLATE
FROSTING

Makes about 4 cups

14 tablespoons refined coconut oil

2 cups evaporated cane sugar

1½ cups unsweetened cocoa powder

1 cup soy creamer

½ teaspoon pure vanilla extract

¼ teaspoon fine sea salt

In a 2- to 3-quart saucepan over medium heat, melt the oil. Stir in sugar and cocoa powder. Gradually stir in creamer. Heat, stirring almost constantly, until mixture is smooth and hot, but not boiling. Remove from heat and stir in vanilla and salt. Set aside to cool to room temperature, until thick enough to spread.

Carrot Cake with Cream Cheese Frosting

Serves 10 to 12

1 cup safflower oil,
  plus more for the pans

3 cups whole wheat pastry flour,
  plus more for the pans

2 cups evaporated cane sugar
  (or other dry sweetener)

2 teaspoons baking powder

2 teaspoons baking soda

2 teaspoons cinnamon

1 teaspoon refined sea salt

2 cups finely shredded carrots
  (about 2 carrots)

2 cups unsweetened applesauce

2 teaspoons vanilla

1½ cups chopped walnuts

4 cups Vegan Cream Cheese
  Frosting (recipe follows)

Preheat oven to 350°F. Oil two 9-inch cake pans and line the bottoms with parchment. Oil the parchment and dust the pans lightly with flour.

In a large bowl, sift together the flour, sugar, baking powder, baking soda, cinnamon, and salt; set aside.

In another large bowl, combine the oil, carrots, applesauce, and vanilla, stirring until smooth. Stir in the flour mixture in 3 or 4 additions, mixing until barely combined. Add walnuts, stirring until just combined.

Transfer the batter to the prepared pans and smooth the surfaces. Bake for 35 to 40 minutes, or until the cakes spring back when lightly touched in the center and begin to pull away from the sides of the pan. Cool on racks for 10 minutes. Unmold the cakes and return to racks to cool thoroughly.

Spread each cake with about ¼ of the Vegan Cream Cheese Frosting. Stack the cakes, then use the remaining frosting to coat the sides of the cake.

VEGAN CREAM CHEESE FROSTING

Makes about 4 cups

12 ounces vegan cream cheese

1 tablespoon pure vanilla extract

¼ teaspoon salt

8 cups (about 2 pounds) powdered evaporated cane sugar (or other dry sweetener)

In the bowl of a stand mixer or in a large bowl with a hand mixer, combine the cream cheese, vanilla, and salt, mixing on medium speed until smooth. With the mixer on low speed, add the sugar, about ½ cup at a time. Increase the speed to high and beat until light and fluffy, 1 to 2 minutes.

Chocolate Cake

Serves 12 to 16

¾ cup safflower oil, plus more
   for the pan

2 cups whole wheat pastry flour

1½ cups evaporated cane sugar

1 tablespoon cream of tartar

2 teaspoons baking soda

½ teaspoon fine sea salt

¾ cup vegan chocolate chips

1¼ cups soy milk

¾ cup unsweetened applesauce

½ tablespoon pure vanilla extract

4 ounces unsweetened vegan
   chocolate, chopped

1 tablespoon apple cider vinegar

2 cups Fudgy Chocolate Frosting
   (see page 171) (optional)

Write out your will while it's
cooking. It's just that good.

Preheat oven to 350°F. Oil a 13 x 9-inch baking pan; set aside.

In a large bowl, sift together the flour, sugar, cream of tartar, baking soda, and salt. Stir in the chocolate chips; set aside.

In a medium bowl, combine the oil, soy milk, applesauce, and vanilla, stirring until smooth; set aside.

In the top of a double boiler or in a medium metal bowl set over a pot of gently simmering water, melt the chocolate, stirring just until smooth.

Add the oil mixture into the flour mixture, stirring until smooth. Add the melted chocolate, stirring until smooth. Stir in the vinegar.

Transfer the batter to the prepared pan and smooth the surface. Bake for 40 to 45 minutes, until the cake springs back when lightly touched in the center and begins to pull away from the sides of the pan. Thoroughly cool on a cooling rack before frosting with Fudgy Chocolate Frosting.

Dream Bars

Makes 16 to 20

1½ cups vegan cookie crumbs
  (see note on page 168)

¼ cup refined coconut oil, melted

⅔ cups raw (turbinado) evaporated
  cane sugar, divided

⅔ cup peanut butter

2 tablespoons water

¼ cup vegan butter

¾ cup vegan chocolate chips

1 cup chopped walnuts

½ cup unsweetened shredded
  coconut

1 (13.5-ounce can) coconut milk

2 tablespoons agave nectar

1 tablespoon arrowroot or 3½
  teaspoons cornstarch dissolved
  into ½ tablespoon water

Preheat oven to 350° F.

In a medium bowl, combine the cookie crumbs, coconut oil, and ⅓ cup of the sugar, stirring until the mixture is uniformly moist. Transfer to a 13 x 9-inch baking pan and press the mixture evenly into the bottom.

Heat the peanut butter in a 1-quart saucepan over medium heat, stirring occasionally, until soft enough to pour. Drizzle the peanut butter over the cookie crumb mixture (don't worry about spreading it—just drizzle it evenly around).

In a 1-quart saucepan over medium heat, combine the remaining ⅓ cup of sugar and the water, stirring occasionally until the sugar is melted. Reduce the heat to low and continue to cook, swirling (not stirring) occasionally, until the mixture is a dark honey color. Remove the saucepan from the heat and swirl in the butter. Presto—you've got butterscotch sauce! Pour the butterscotch sauce evenly over the peanut butter. Top with chocolate chips, walnuts, and coconut, sprinkling each evenly.

In a small bowl, whisk together the coconut milk, agave, and arrowroot mixture. Pour the coconut milk mixture evenly over the toppings and bake for 30 minutes, until the coconut milk is set and the edges are browned. Thoroughly cool on a cooling rack before cutting into squares. For best results, set aside at room temperature overnight or in the refrigerator for 1 or 2 hours before serving.

Don't plan on sharing these with anyone. Hoard them for yourself.

Rice Pudding

Serves 4 to 6

2 cups soy creamer (or 1
   13.5-ounce can coconut
   milk plus ⅓ cup water)

1 cup water

1 cup medium-grain brown rice

Pinch fine sea salt

⅔ cup raisins, golden raisins,
   or a combination (optional)

2 tablespoons agave nectar

½ teaspoon pure vanilla extract

¼ teaspoon ground cinnamon

In a 2-quart saucepan over high heat, combine 1 cup of the creamer or coconut milk mixture, the water, rice, and salt. Bring to a boil, reduce the heat to a simmer, cover, and cook until the water is absorbed and the rice is almost tender, about 40 minutes.

Stir in the remaining 1 cup of creamer or coconut milk mixture, the raisins (if using), agave, vanilla, and cinnamon. Bring to a simmer and cook, stirring occasionally, until the raisins are plump and the rice is tender, about 5 minutes.

Spoon the pudding into bowls and let cool. Serve at room temperature or cover and refrigerate for about an hour before serving chilled.

If the pudding seems too thick, which can be the case if it's served cold, you can stir in a little soy milk or creamer.

Fresh Fruit Crisp

½ cup refined coconut oil,
  plus more for the pan

1 cup plus 2 tablespoons Sucanat,
  (or other dry sweetener)

½ cup plus 1 tablespoon whole
  wheat pastry flour

½ cup rolled oats

¾ teaspoon salt

1 teaspoon ground cinnamon

8 cups cored or pitted fresh fruit,
  one type or a combination,
  thinly sliced

2 tablespoons lemon juice

1 teaspoon pure vanilla extract

1 pint vegan vanilla ice cream
  (optional)

Preheat oven to 375°F. Oil an 8 x 8-inch baking pan.

In a medium bowl, combine 1 cup of the Sucanat, ½ cup of the flour, the oats, and ½ teaspoon of the salt. Using a pastry cutter or your fingertips, cut in the oil, mixing until the biggest pieces are the size of peas; set aside.

In a large bowl, combine the remaining 2 tablespoons of Sucanat, 1 tablespoon of flour, ¼ teaspoon of salt, and the cinnamon. Mix in the fruit, lemon juice, and vanilla.

Transfer the fruit to the prepared baking dish, spreading it evenly. Sprinkle on the topping. Bake for 30 minutes. If the fruit isn't yet tender (baking time will depend on the type of fruit), cover lightly with foil and bake for an additional 20 or 30 minutes.

Serve warm or at room temperature, topped with vegan vanilla ice cream, if using.

For the fresh fruit, use whatever is in season—whatever's the most ripe and full-flavored. Make it with apples in the fall, berries in the spring, and peaches in the summer. Apples will take the longer cooking time, pears a little less, and most other fruit will be done in 40 minutes—varying a little depending on ripeness and how thinly the fruit is sliced. Peeling isn't necessary.

After-Dinner Mint

Food is the fuel that keeps us going. It supplies our bodies with energy and sustenance and literally makes life possible. But it's also so much more than that. It's the gateway to paradise. A gift from the heavens. Life's greatest pleasure. Every time we eat, we have the capacity to experience unparalleled ecstasy. Multiple times a day. So why do people forget to eat? Or eat standing up? Or grab something quick? Hell, it beats the shit out of us. We never do that stuff—we friggin' love eating more than anything else in the world. And we bask in the glory of every bite we take.

Eating is like a religious experience. And every meal is like an offering to your temple. So like you would for any place of worship, have reverence for your body. You shouldn't put garbage in your mouth any sooner than you'd go to church wearing crotchless panties. Now granted, sometimes you wear less than your Sunday best to church, and that's fine—God loves you, anyway. And sometimes you eat less than your best, and that's okay, too. But you wouldn't make a habit of dressing like crap for church and you shouldn't make a habit of eating crap, either.

We each get one body to last us an entire lifetime. And more than any other factor, food affects how well and for how long this body will serve us. So if you didn't care before, start caring now. Take the time to learn which foods are healthy and which aren't. And take the time to start enjoying everything you eat. Doing "it" standing up and "quickies" are for sex, not eating. So slow down, pick out a recipe, and sit down to a nice meal tonight. After dinner, you can have a quickie.

GLOSSARY

We know that for many of you, this is a whole new way of eating. So we salute your willingness to take it on—change is definitely hard. But it doesn't have to be scary. The more you know, the less intimidated you'll be. Knowledge is power.

Having said that, behold the glossary. (If there's an ingredient you're curious about that we don't define . . . look it up in a dictionary or online. Don't be a Needy Bitch.)

....

Agave Nectar or Syrup: A sweetener, similar to honey, that comes from the Agave plant (where tequila happens to come from, too). It's less refined than regular sugar, so it doesn't contain processing chemicals. Buy the "raw" version.

Arrowroot: A starch flour made from the root of a plant. Like cornstarch, it's used as a thickener.

Bacon (vegan): Bacon alternative made from soy protein, wheat gluten, and other ingredients. Tastes like friggin' bacon, but doesn't encompass slaughtering a pig.

Bragg's Liquid Amino Acids: Tastes kinda like soy sauce, but contains no MSG. Made from soybeans and purified water. A must have with steamed-veggies and brown rice. Use Bragg's instead of soy sauce.

Cheese (vegan): A dairy-free cheese substitute that contains no milk, rennet (an enzyme from the stomach lining of calves), no casein (a milk protein), no whey (the liquid portion of milk that has curdled), and no other gross-out factor. Our favorite brand is Follow Your Heart.

Ener-G Egg Replacer: A vegan replacement for eggs in baking. Made from potato starch and tapioca flour to mimic eggs in recipes. Comes in powder form; just mix with water.

Evaporated Cane Sugar: Made from sugar cane, only the water has been removed. It's less processed than regular sugar, so it retains some nutrients.

Kelp Powder: Granules made from seaweed that lend a mild salty and/ or fishy flavor to dishes.

Mayonnaise (vegan): A dairy-, egg-, and cholesterol-free mayonnaise substitute. Our favorite brand: Follow Your Heart Vegenaise.

Nutritional Yeast Flakes: A non-leavening yeast that has a cheesy flavor. A food supplement that contains B vitamins and tastes great on salads, pizzas, and popcorn!

Oil (Coconut, Flaxseed, Hempseed): There is so much conflicting information regarding oils and there are so many different schools of thought. Here's the one we subscribe to: Oils are best when kept intact and not heated. So when you're using oil as a dressing or to add flavor to something after it's cooked, unrefined oil is best. If you can stand the taste, flaxseed oil is really good for you. Hempseed oil, cold-pressed extra virgin olive oil, and sesame seed oil are all good options, too. Heating oils, especially at high temperatures, can alter them into harmful toxic substances. However, a girl's gotta eat, and sometimes a girl's gotta heat her oil. With that said, some oils withstand heat better than others. Refined coconut oil is the best oil for high heat cooking. Canola oil and safflower oil are other decent options. (Never continue to use oil that has burnt or is smoking. And never save and re-use oil that you've already cooked with. Re-used fryer oil is just one of the reasons fast food is so damn bad for you.)

Parmesan (vegan): A Parmesan cheese substitute that is made without any dairy components. (Some companies make it with a soy-based version, and others make it with nutritional yeast and nuts.)

Pasta: Substitute regular, refined, white pasta with whole wheat, brown rice, or quinoa pasta. These are healthier alternatives that contain nutrients and fiber.

Rice Milk: Dairy-, lactose-, and cholesterol-free milk alternative made from brown rice, water, and a small amount of brown rice sweetener.

Seitan: High-protein meat substitute made from wheat gluten. The texture may freak you out at first, but keep trying it. Soon, you'll be hooked.

Soy Butter: A dairy-free butter substitute usually made from a blend of oils. Be sure to get the non-hydrogenated kind.

Soy Milk: Dairy-, lactose-, and cholesterol-free milk alternative made from soybeans. High in protein, vitamins, and minerals.

Sucanat: Sugar in its most natural form: SUgar CAne NATural. It's extracted from unrefined sugar cane where only the water has been removed. It retains the molasses, as well as the vitamins and minerals.

Tahini: Thick paste made from ground sesame seeds.

Tempeh: A vegan, meat-like alternative made from fermented soybeans. High in protein. The texture isn't really meaty—it's more nutty and grainy, kinda. Just shut up and try it.

Textured Soy Protein (also known as texturized vegetable protein): A meat substitute made from defatted soy flour that's compressed and processed into bite-size chunks. Generally, it needs to be rehydrated with water when using.

Tofu: Made from processed soybean curds. Good source of calcium and protein. Cholesterol-free, baby. Tofu is a total chameleon in recipes and can take on whatever flavor you want. It does take getting used to.

Turbinado: Made from 100 percent sugar cane. It's what's left after raw sugar has been washed, allowing the natural molasses to remain.

Vegan (noun): A person who abstains from eating cows, chickens, pigs, fish, eggs, and dairy. "I am a vegan."

Vegan (adjective): 1. The state of being with regard to not eating cows, chickens, pigs, fish, eggs, and dairy. "I am vegan." 2. A product free of animal ingredients. "Is that cookie vegan?"

Metric Conversion Tips

For all you bitches who use the metric system . . .

Generic Formulas for Metric Conversion

Ounces to grams	multiply ounces by 28.35
Pounds to grams	multiply pounds by 453.5
Cups to liters	multiply cups by .24
Fahrenheit to Centigrade	subtract 32 from Fahrenheit, multiply by five and divide by 9

Oven Temperatures

Degrees Fahrenheit	Degrees Centigrade	British Gas Marks
200°	93°	—
250°	120°	—
275°	140°	1
300°	150°	2
325°	165°	3
350°	175°	4
375°	190°	5
400°	200°	6
450°	230°	8

Metric Equivalents for Volume

U.S.	Imperial	Metric
1/8 tsp.	—	0.6 ml
1/2 tsp.	—	2.5 ml
3/4 tsp.	—	4.0 ml
1 tsp.	—	5.0 ml
1 1/2 tsp.	—	7.0 ml
2 tsp.	—	10.0 ml
3 tsp.	—	15.0 ml
4 tsp.	—	20.0 ml
1 Tbsp.	—	15.0 ml
1 1/2 Tbsp.	—	22.0 ml
2 Tbsp. (1/8 cup)	1 fl. oz	30.0 ml
2 1/2 Tbsp.	—	37.0 ml
3 Tbsp.	—	44.0 ml
1/8 cup	—	57.0 ml
4 Tbsp. (1/4 cup)	2 fl. oz	59.0 ml
5 Tbsp.	—	74.0 ml
6 Tbsp.	—	89.0 ml
8 Tbsp. (1/2 cup)	4 fl. oz	120.0 ml
3/4 cup	6 fl. oz	178.0 ml
1 cup	8 fl. oz	237.0 ml
(.24 liters)		
1 1/2 cups	—	354.0 ml
1 3/4 cups	—	414.0 ml
2 cups (1 pint)	16 fl. oz	473.0 ml
4 cups (1 quart)	32 fl. oz	(.95 liters)
5 cups	—	(1.183 liters)
16 cups (1 gallon)	128 fl. oz	(3.8 liters)

Metric Equivalents for Weight

U.S.	Metric
1 oz	28 g
2 oz	58 g
3 oz	85 g
4 oz (¼ lb.)	113 g
5 oz	142 g
6 oz	170 g
7 oz	199 g
8 oz (½ lb.)	227 g
10 oz	284 g
12 oz (¾ lb.)	340 g
14 oz	397 g
16 oz (1 lb.)	454 g

Metric Equivalents for Butter

U.S.	Metric
2 tsp.	10.0 g
1 Tbsp.	15.0 g
1½ Tbsp.	22.5 g
2 Tbsp. (1 oz)	55.0 g
3 Tbsp.	70.0 g
¼ lb. (1 stick)	110.0 g
½ lb. (2 sticks)	220.0 g

Metric Equivalents for Length

(USE ALSO FOR PAN SIZES)

··

U.S.	Metric
¼ inch	.65 cm
½ inch	1.25 cm
1 inch	2.50 cm
2 inches	5.00 cm
3 inches	6.00 cm
4 inches	8.00 cm
5 inches	11.00 cm
6 inches	15.00 cm
7 inches	18.00 cm
8 inches	20.00 cm
9 inches	23.00 cm
12 inches	30.50 cm
15 inches	38.00 cm

INDEX

Skinny Bitch

Skinny Bitch

*A no-nonsense, tough-love guide for
savvy girls who want to stop eating crap
and start looking fabulous!*

by Rory Freedman and Kim Barnouin

Running Press
PHILADELPHIA • LONDON

Library of Congress Control Number 2005901966

ISBN: 978-0-7624-3541-8

Cover and interior designed by Maria Taffera Lewis
Typography: Bauer Bodoni and Dutch 801

This book may be ordered by mail from the publisher.
Please include $2.50 for postage and handling.
But try your bookstore first!

Running Press Book Publishers
2300 Chestnut Street
Philadelphia, Pennsylvania 19103

Visit us on the web!
www.runningpress.com
www.skinnybitch.net

Contents

Dedication

For Tony Robbins and Dr. Wayne Dyer,
with much love and appreciation.
It is because of your work that this book exists.

And for all the truth-speakers and seekers who have made
the world a better place while dramatically influencing our lives:
We thank you and honor all that you have done
and continue to do in the name of what is right.

Namastè.

Acknowledgments

It is with the utmost gratitude that we thank Lyssie Lakatos, Tammy Lakatos-Shames, Talia Cohen, Laura Dail, Jennifer Kasius, Maria Taffera Lewis, Nancy Armstrong, Margarete Gockel, and Greg Jones for bringing this book to life.
We acknowledge the keen eyes of Meri Freedman and Dr. Amy Joy Lanou, and heartfelt thanks to our dream-team: Jon Anderson, Craig Herman, Seta Zink, Peter Costanzo, and everyone at Perseus Books, Running Press and Creative Artists Agency for leading us above and beyond.

For your kind and patient help, we sincerely thank Chloe Jo Berman, James Costa, Matt Green, Bruce Friedrich, Holly Sternberg, Mark Gold, Kristina Johnson, Sara Chenoweth, Harold Brown, Ryan Zinn, Michele Simon, Talia Berman, Danielle Simon, Wayne Pacelle, Jay and Wendy Baxter, and Shaun Zaken.
We are honored by the generous contributions of C. David Coates, Christine Hoza Farlow, D.C., and Tim VanOrden and cannot thank you enough.

Rory:

Kim, my partner in crime, I cannot imagine the existence I'd be leading if we never met. Thank you for changing the course of my life and enlightening me with your glow. You had me at hello.

It is with true adoration that I thank Tracy Silverman, who started me on this path, Lauren Silverman, who inspired me to commit to it more fully, Jesse Hildebrandt, for enabling me to do so, and my magical friends who made the journey by my side: Sue Foley, Todd and Lisa Adamek, Nora Ariffin, Emily Ashba, Dave Feeney, Fara Horowitz, Jill Iacuzzo, Jessica Jonas, Margaret Klinger, Denise Kunisch, Lisa Leder, Chris Lucia, Julie Lundberg, Kerri Meyers, Lori Morgen, Luke Orefice, Michelle Pappas, Andrea Pendas, Brian and MC Permenter, Jackie Poper, Randie Rolantz, Christine Santoro, Kim Snowden, Nora Stein, Louie and Christine Tibolla, Susan Weinberg, and all my PR pals who are too numerous to name.

To my grandmothers, Florence Freedman and Frances Levine, thank you for your inexhaustible supplies of love and faith. For your endless enthusiasm and loving encouragement, I thank my sister and brother-in-law, Lesley and Tim Bailey. Most of all, my parents, Rick and Meri Freedman— it is with an overflowing heart that I thank you for a lifetime of your unwavering support and love.

Kim:

My amazing friend and business partner, Rory,
without you none of this would be happening. I thank God every day
that we met and shared the same dream. We leapt
and the net appeared. Thank you for leaping with me.

Keesha Whitehurst Frederickson, I am so glad you are a part
of my life. Thank you for all the laughter and love,
and for being so special.

To all my other friends who honor me
with their day-to-day presence, I thank you.

A million thanks to my wonderful parents,
Richard and Linda Robinson, who believed in me and cheered me
on through the hard times and the good times.

To Jeri, Chrissy, Amanda, Melissa, Alex, and Elliot: I love you!

And last but not least, my love: my husband, Stephane.
There are not enough words in any language to express my love for
you. I am so grateful for your never-ending patience,
constant faith, pure love, and undying support.
I feel so blessed to be traveling through this life with you.
Je T'aime.

Introduction

Are you sick and tired of being fat? Good. If you can't take one more day of self-loathing, you're ready to get skinny. You don't need a degree in biology to get skinny. You don't need to starve yourself to get skinny. You don't need to spend all day at the gym to get skinny. You just need to smarten up and use your head. Really. It is that simple. We have been so brainwashed by fad diets, magazine articles, and advertising that we have forgotten how to think for ourselves.

Skinny Bitch delivers the truth about food, so that you can make intelligent and educated decisions for yourself. This knowledge will empower you to become a skinny bitch.

This is not a diet. This is a way of life. A way to enjoy food. A way to feel healthy, clean, energized and pure. It's time to reclaim your mind and body. It's time to strut your skinny ass down the street like you're in an episode of *Charlie's Angels* with some really cool song playing in the background. It's time to prance around in a thong like you rule the world. It's time to get skinny.

Chapter 1
Give It Up

O kay. Use your head. You need to get healthy if you want to get skinny. Healthy = skinny. Unhealthy = fat. The first thing you need to do is give up your gross vices. Don't act surprised! You cannot keep eating the same shit and expect to get skinny. Or smoke. So don't even try some pathetic excuse like, "But if I quit smoking, I'll gain weight." No one wants to hear it. Cigarettes are for losers. They are so 1989 and totally uncool. Not only do they screw up your whole body chemistry, but they also kill your taste buds. It's no wonder you eat shit and garbage. Smoking's out. Give it up.

Of course it's easier to socialize after you've had a few drinks. But being a fat pig will hinder you, sober or drunk. And habitual drinking equals fat-pig syndrome. Beer is for frat boys, not skinny bitches. It makes you fat, bloated, and farty. Why do you think when kids go away to college they gain the "freshman fifteen"? Beer, duh. Alcohol isn't any better. It raises the level of hydrochloric acid in your stomach, wreaking havoc on the digestive process. If you suffer from poor digestion, then your food will not pass through your body properly. Hence, bloated fat-pig syndrome. To make matters worse, some alcohol (and non-organic wines) still contains urethane, a cancer-causing chemical.[1] To boot, both beer and alcohol jack up your blood-sugar levels, which is bad for your bod. And don't kid yourself: When you have a hangover, you're bound to eat shit all day long. Trade your booze for organic red wine produced without sulfites. (Sulfites are additives—used in food and wine—to extend shelf life and fight bacteria growth. Asthma and allergic reactions can be triggered by sulfites. Even if wine is organic, that doesn't mean it is produced without sulfites. Read the label; it should say "No Sulfites Added" or "NSA." Frey Vineyards makes organic, sulfite-free wines.) This magical elixir—organic red wine with NSA—is rich in cancer-fighting antioxidants, can reduce risk of stroke, helps thin the blood, and has flavonoids, which lower cholesterol. Yes, organic red wine is good for you. No, you should not drink a bottle by yourself every day. Alcohol abuse can cause infertility, cancer, infectious diseases, cardiovascular disease, shrinking of the cerebral cortex, and alter brain-cell function. If you need help quitting drinking, call the Alcoholics Anonymous World Headquarters at (212) 870-3400 to find an AA meeting near you, or visit www.alcoholics-anonymous.org.

Brace yourselves, girls: Soda is liquid Satan. It is the devil. It is garbage. There is nothing in soda that should be put into your body. For starters, soda's high levels of phosphorous can increase calcium loss from the body, as can its sodium and caffeine. [Cousens, *Conscious Eating*, 475] You know what this means—bone loss, which may lead to osteoporosis. And the last time we checked, sugar, found in soda by the boatload, does not make you skinny! Now don't go patting yourself on the back if you drink diet soda. That stuff is even worse. Aspartame (an ingredient commonly found in diet sodas and other sugar-free foods) has been blamed for a slew of scary maladies, like arthritis, birth defects, fibromyalgia, Alzheimer's, lupus, multiple sclerosis, and diabetes.[2] When methyl alcohol, a component of aspartame, enters your body, it turns into formaldehyde. Formaldehyde is toxic and carcinogenic (cancer-causing).[3] Laboratory scientists use formaldehyde as a disinfectant or preservative. They don't fucking *drink* it. Perhaps you have a lumpy ass because you are preserving your fat cells with diet soda. The Food and Drug Administration (FDA) has received more complaints about aspartame than any other ingredient to date.[4] Want more bad news? When aspartame is paired with carbs, it causes your brain to slow down its production of serotonin.[5] A healthy level of serotonin is needed to be happy and well balanced. So drinking soda can make you fat, sick, and unhappy.

Unless you're from Mars, you've heard about the "eight glasses of water a day" thing. If you're filling up on 16 ounces of liquid Satan at a time, chances are you're not getting your 64 ounces of water a day. Water is vital for keeping your body clean and detoxified. It literally flushes out all the shit and toxins your body stores from your horrendous diet. You might be fat because you don't poop enough. Drinking lots of water can help with the elimination process. If the taste of water bores you, try jazzing up the flavor with a slice of lemon or lime, or, if you're feeling sassy, toss in a strawberry or raspberry. Say goodbye to soda and hello to a sweet ass.

"Don't talk to me until I've had my morning coffee." Uhm . . . *pathetic*! Coffee is for pussies. Think about how widely accepted it has become that people *need* coffee to wake up. You should not *need* anything to wake up. If you can't wake up without it, it's because you are either addicted to caffeine, sleep deprived, or a generally unhealthy slob. It may seem like the end of the world to give up your daily dose, especially if you rely on Starbucks as a good place to meet men. But it's not heroin, girls, and you'll learn to live without it. Caffeine can cause headaches, digestive problems, irritation of the stomach and bladder, peptic ulcers, diarrhea, constipation, fatigue, anxiety, and depression. It affects every organ system, from the nervous system to the skin. Caffeine raises stress hormone levels, inhibits important enzyme systems that are responsible for cleaning the body, and sensitizes nerve reception sites.[6] One study even links caffeine to an increased susceptibility to diabetes.[7] But don't go grabbing for the decaf. Coffee, whether regular or decaf, is highly acidic.[8] Acidic foods cause your body to produce fat cells, in order to keep the acid away from your organs.[9] (Please, do not link this acid issue to citrus and other fruits. We discuss this in depth later on page 38.) So coffee equals fat cells. P.S. It also makes your breath smell like ass. Furthermore, coffee beans, like other crops, are grown with chemical pesticides. One insecticide, D-D-7, has been banned in the United States, but is still used by other countries from which we import coffee beans.[10] So every single morning, you are starting your day with a dose of poison. Add sugar or other artificial sweeteners, top it off with milk or cream, and you'll be fat forever. If you enjoy an occasional cup of coffee, fine. But if you need it, give it up.

A much better way to start the day is with a cup of caffeine-free herbal tea—organic, of course. Decaffeinated green tea is like a wonder drug. Its anti-aging and antibacterial qualities are as renowned as its reputation for fighting cancer, combating allergies, and lowering blood pressure. Go to a coffeehouse, if you must. Just get a decaf organic herbal tea instead of coffee. Miss your caffeine jolt? Get a fresh-squeezed organic juice for an instant jumpstart. Once you are rid of your caffeine addiction, you will get totally high from fresh-squeezed juice.

Junk food will never go away. It becomes more alluring by the minute with laboratory-developed aromas, artificial flavors, chemical food colors, toxic preservatives, and heart-stopping hydrogenated oils. We know these are all impossible to resist, but no one ever got skinny on junk food. Use your head. Candy bars, potato chips, and ice cream taste like heaven, of course. But they will pitch a tent on your hips and camp out all year. Not only are they bogged down with saturated fats, sugars, hydrogenated oils, calories, and cholesterol, but they also contain enough chemical residues to put hair on your chest. Ever heard of butylated hydroxyamisole (BHA) or butylated hydroxytoluene (BHT)? Most people haven't, even though these chemical preservatives are either put in food or into the packaging.[11] The FDA doesn't require companies to divulge the presence of these beauties if they are used in packaging, though they can come into contact with the food you're eating. So your junk food has a shelf life of twenty-two years and will probably outlive your fat, sorry ass. Now before you decide you're so smart because you only buy fat-free snacks, get a hold of yourself. Whenever you see the words "fat-free" or "low-fat," think of the words "chemical shit storm." Read the ingredients. Do you really think sugar or hydrogenated oils or eggs or milk won't make you fat? Sober up, asshole. By the way, sugar, like coffee, creates an acidic environment in your body.[12] You just learned that acidic foods cause your body to produce fat cells. So you do the math: sugar = fat. If you'd drag your cankles to a health food store, you'd find aisle after aisle of "acceptable junk food." Guilt-free garbage that tastes so good, you'll do naked cartwheels around your living room. We are not saying you have to give up junk food to get skinny. You just have to trade your old junk food for new junk food. In Chapter 11, we provide an "acceptable junk food" list that'll make your nipples hard.

Are you a pill popper? Do you reach for over-the-counter medicine for every sniffle, sneeze, ache, and pain? Toughen up. Our bodies, when properly cared for, function as perfect machines. Our brains tell us when something is wrong by giving us pain or discomfort. When we pop pills to rid this "dis-ease," we are masking the symptoms without resolving the problem. Every time you take medicine, you interfere with your body's natural ability to heal itself. You are alleviating those intelligent responses that alert you to a problem, and sending false signals to your brain. If you have a headache, you might be tired, dehydrated, or suffering from a minor food allergy. Most likely, your body is having an adverse reaction to the unhealthy crap you're eating. Taking two aspirin is not the answer. If your nose is running, your body is trying to rid itself of something through your snot. But you, drama queen, take cold medicine to stop your booger flow. Now you've gone and fucked up everything. Medicine is made of chemicals. Never mind that the Food and Drug Administration gives meds their stamp of approval. They also allow the use of aspartame. Use your own damn brain. Do you think putting *chemicals* in your body is good for you? Every medicine comes complete with a list of side effects. That means that taking medicine will make you feel better for the moment, but will fuck up something else in your body. Yeah, getting cramps totally sucks. It's supposed to. Every month you endure cramps (without medication), you are preparing for the physical pain of childbirth. So suck it up. Stop interfering with Mother Nature.

(Obviously, if you are on prescribed medication, you need to consult a physician before discontinuing it.)

Give up the notion that you can be sedentary and still lose weight. You need to exercise, you lazy shit. Eating properly will dramatically improve your health, body, and all aspects of your life. But you've still gotta move your ass. Anyone with a brain can do the math: When done in conjunction with a good diet, exercise will make you lose weight faster than healthy eating alone. You don't need to spend seven days a week at the gym. In fact, you shouldn't, because too much exercise is bad for you. It can lead to dehydration, arthritis, osteoporosis, and injuries like strains, sprains, and fractures. Over-exercising can also cause low body-fat levels, which can disrupt the menstrual cycle and cause reproductive problems.[13] You want to be a Skinny Bitch, not a scrawny bitch. Twenty minutes of cardiovascular a day, five days a week, is a good starting point. Then, after a couple of weeks, kick it up a notch. Depending on your fitness goals, you can increase your cardiovascular workout or add strength training to your routine. Aim for working out in the morning, if you can. When we exercise, our elevated heart rates and deep breathing cause our "bodyminds" to enter a fat-burning mode that can last throughout the day.[14] Regardless of what time you work out, you'll soon become addicted to exercising. When we are active enough to break a sweat, our brains release endorphins and feel-good opiates. Exercise burns fat and calories, improves circulation, regulates crapping, defines muscles, builds strength, and detoxifies the body through sweating. Plus, working out tends to keep our junk food cravings and elephant appetites at bay. It's a win-win. Work out.

Chapter 2
Carbs: The Truth

Never before has the United States seen such a ridiculous diet trend as the "low-carb" phenomenon. Every restaurant, grocery store, and fast-food chain caters to this utter nonsense. Even soda and beer companies have spent millions developing and marketing low-carb drinks. Everyone has jumped on the bandwagon, hoping to capitalize on the trend, whether it is healthy or not. Not.

Carbohydrates are compounds made up of carbon, hydrogen,

and oxygen, and they are *vital* for providing energy for our bodies
and brains. Without them, we would be comatose zombies. When
we eat food, our bodies turn the carbohydrates into glucose for
immediate energy and the rest is stored as glycogen for reserves.

Yet all carbs are not created equal. There are two types: simple
and complex. Simple carbohydrates suck and are as nutritionally
beneficial as toilet paper. They are mostly made up of sugar, which
releases too quickly, almost violently, into our bodies, causing
"sugar highs" and then "crashes." This tends to leave us feeling
hungry, so we eat more. On the other hand, complex carbohydrates
are comprised of starch and fiber and release gradually, providing a
steady source of energy. They make us feel full and satisfied and
are easily broken down to release their energy. Shitty simple carbohydrates include white flour, white pasta (durum semolina), white
rice, and white sugar. These are the bad boys that give all carbs a
bad reputation. For some asinine reason, food manufacturers
decided that we wouldn't buy their products unless they were white
and soft. So they took natural grains, like brown rice and whole
wheat, and stripped away all their nutrients, vitamins, and minerals
to achieve the color and texture change. This refining process totally

compromises the nutritional integrity of the food—all for appearances. So companies then add these nutrients back into their refined, milled foods and use terms like "enriched" or "fortified." But there's no use trying to fool with Mother Nature. Our bodies cannot absorb these added-in minerals with the same ease.[15] Tragically, most cereals, pastas, rice, bagels, breads, cookies, muffins, cakes, and pastries have been bastardized in this manner. Pay attention to how your body feels when you eat these foods. Chances are you'll notice moderate to severe mood swings and energy surges and losses.

Fear not. There are so many complex carbohydrates (Mother Nature is generous) that you'll never miss the simple shit. Bask in the glory of potatoes, yams, sweet potatoes, barley, corn, brown rice, beans, hummus, lentils, quinoa (a grain, pronounced KEEN-wa), millet, and pasta made from brown rice, whole wheat, or vegetables. Bionaturae, Ancient Harvest, Eddie's Spaghetti, Lundberg Farms, Westbrae, Pastariso, and DeBoles Organic all carry these "good carb" pastas. Relish the beauty of breads and cookies and muffins made from whole wheat and other whole grains. (Whole grains are any that haven't been bleached, stripped, or refined and still possess all the nutrients from the original grain.) Food For Life has an amazing line of whole and sprouted grain breads, and Pacific Bakery and French Meadow Bakery carry organic breads that aren't too shabby, either. Don't forget the bounty of vegetables and fruits—complex carbs that supply the body with vitamins, minerals, and fiber.

Yeah, you heard us—fruit. Eat it. The most irritating thing about the low-carb craze is the resistance to eating fruit. Fruit is, quite possibly, the most perfect food in existence. It is unique in that it barely requires any work to be digested. High in enzymes, it effortlessly passes through the body, supplying carbohydrates, fiber, vitamins, minerals, fatty acids, amino acids, and cancer-fighting tannins and flavonoids. Because it is made up of mostly water, fruit hydrates the body and aids in cleansing, detoxifying, and eliminating.

Best-selling *Fit for Life* authors Harvey and Marilyn Diamond found that fruit best serves our bodies when eaten alone because it is so easily and quickly digested. When we eat fruit with other foods, it cannot pass through our bodies as quickly. So it rots and ferments in our stomachs. This can cause burping, bloating, and heartburn. To combat this, the Diamonds recommend eating fruit on an empty stomach, first meal of the day, and waiting thirty minutes before eating anything else.[16] (We know this will be tough for some people, and it's okay if you aren't ready to tackle this challenge yet. It's just an ideal to aim for.)

So shout it from the rooftops until every one of your dumb-ass, misinformed friends hears: YOU CAN EAT BREAD AND FRUIT!

Chapter 3

Sugar is the Devil

W e all know how difficult it is to stay away from sugar. But if you don't exorcise this demon from your diet, you will never be a skinny bitch. Take a look around your kitchen and become aware of all the places the devil is lurking. Probably in places you wouldn't ever expect to find "him." Read the ingredients of your breakfast cereals, breads, crackers, junk foods, everything. Sugar is like crack, and food manufacturers know that if they add it to their products, you'll keep coming back for more.

What is this evil entity? In its simplest form, it is the juice from a sugar cane plant. A plant—that seems benign, right? And it is, in moderation, ingested in its raw, simplest form. But all the enzymes, fiber, vitamins, and minerals are destroyed during the refining process.[17] First, the cane is pressed to extract the juice. Then, the juice is boiled so that it will thicken and crystallize. Next, it is centrifuged, or spun, to remove the syrup. After that, the sugar is washed and filtered to remove any nonsugar materials and to decolorize it. (By the way, sugar filters are commonly made of charred animal bones. Nasty.) Finally, the sugar is dried and packaged. So you see, refined sugar has no nutritional value. And it's usually in foods that contain gobs of fat, lots of useless calories, and loads of cholesterol. So, you become addicted to foods (because they contain sugar) that have a large amount of fat, saturated fat, hydrogenated oils, and calories. Refined sugar, a simple carbohydrate, has been linked to hypoglycemia, yeast overgrowth (check your undies), a weakened immune system, hyperactivity, attention deficit disorder, enlargement of the liver and kidneys, increase of uric acid in the blood, mental and emotional disorders, dental cavi-

ties, and an imbalance of neurotransmitters in the brain.[18] In addition, refined sugars make you *fat*. Excess amounts are stored in the
liver as glycogen. But when the liver is too full, the excess amounts
are returned to the bloodstream as fatty acids.[19] Guess where those
end up? Hips, stomach, thighs, and ass.

The sugar industry is big business in America. The United States
is the largest supplier of sugar-laden foods in the world. It's not
enough to poison our own citizens. We have to fuck up the rest of
the world, too, for a dime.

High fructose corn syrup is another badass that finds its way into
tons of foods. Manufacturers love its versatility and put it in nearly
everything: juice, soda, beer, yogurt, energy bars, cookies, candies,
breads, even frozen goods. High fructose corn syrup is processed
more than sugar and is even sweeter. But it's a friend of the farmer
because it's so cheap to produce. Like refined sugar, it has a negative, dramatic effect on our blood-sugar levels. According to studies
conducted by the *American Journal of Clinical Nutrition,* diabetes
and obesity are directly linked to eating refined sugar and high
fructose corn syrup.[20]

We aren't telling you to give up cookies for the rest of your lives;

we certainly don't want to start a riot. We're simply suggesting that you substitute natural, healthier alternatives for refined sugar. At the top of the list is agave nectar or syrup. This high-nutrient sweetener can actually be beneficial to your health. It doesn't contain any processing chemicals, and the raw version (completely unprocessed) contains vitamins and minerals. Because it absorbs slowly into the bloodstream, agave nectar doesn't have a significant impact on blood-sugar levels. It can be used in place of sugar in any product or recipe.

Stevia, another winner, is derived from a plant found in Paraguay. The Japanese have been using this wonder sweetener for decades, South Americans for centuries. In fact, it is used by hundreds of millions of people around the world to balance blood-sugar levels, reduce cravings for sweets, and aid in digestion. Additionally, it is known for its antimicrobial properties (it inhibits the growth of bacteria). Unfortunately, however, it is the most unrecognized sweetener in the United States. This natural, herbal sweetener contains no calories, has no glycemic index (meaning it won't alter blood sugar), and is even safe for diabetics. But for reasons unknown to intelligent species everywhere, the Food and Drug

Administration won't approve Stevia for use in food products.[21] Maybe they are sleeping with the sugar industry.

Other good substitutes for refined sugar include evaporated cane juice, Sucanat, brown rice syrup, barley malt syrup, Rapadura sugar, Turbinado sugar, raw sugar, beet sugar, date sugar, maple syrup, molasses, and blackstrap molasses. (Some companies add lard to maple syrup or molasses to reduce foaming, so be sure you are buying 100 percent pure, organic products.) Don't shit and piss yourselves, but all of these natural sweeteners possess one or more of the following health benefits: enzymes, calcium, iron, potassium, protein, the B vitamins, magnesium, chromium, fiber, and folic acid. Some even contain complex carbohydrates.[22] We're not saying you should eat naturally sweetened cupcakes three meals a day. We're just saying that you *can* have your cake and eat it. Just use your head regarding the amount of sweets you consume.

A drum roll, please, for a few of our favorite sweets: Uncle Eddie's vegan cookies, Tropical Source or Terra Nostra chocolate bars, Oreo knock-offs by Back to Nature or Country Choice, organic Fig Newmans, and all the cookies by the Sun Flour Baking Co. and the Alternative Baking Co.

Now that you've heard the good news about natural sweeteners, it's time to give up the all the bad ones. Obviously, refined sugar is bad for you, as is high fructose corn syrup. And in case you had your head up your ass during Chapter 1, STOP EATING AND DRINKING PRODUCTS THAT CONTAIN ASPARTAME! This includes diet sodas and sugar-free foods that have NutraSweet or Equal.

When aspartame was put before the FDA for approval, it was denied *eight* times. G.D. Searle, founder of aspartame, tried to get FDA approval in 1973. Clearly, he wasn't bothered by reports from neuroscientist Dr. John Olney and researcher Ann Reynolds (hired by Searle himself) that aspartame was dangerous. Dr. Martha Freeman, a scientist from the FDA Division of Metabolic and Endocrine Drug Products, declared, "The information submitted for review is inadequate to permit a scientific evaluation of clinical safety." Freeman recommended that until the safety of aspartame was proven, marketing the product should not be permitted. Alas, her recommendations were ignored. Somehow, in 1974, Searle got approval to use aspartame in dry foods. However, it wasn't smooth sailing from there. In 1975, the FDA put together a task force to review Searle's testing methods. Task force team leader Phillip

Brodsky said he "had never seen anything as bad as Searle's testing" and called test results "manipulated." Before aspartame
actually made it into dry foods, Olney and attorney and consumer
advocate Jim Turner filed objections against the approval.[23]

In 1977, the FDA asked the U.S. attorney's office to start grand
jury proceedings against Searle for "knowingly misrepresenting
findings and concealing material facts and making false statements
in aspartame safety tests." Shortly after, the U.S. attorney leading
the investigation against Searle was offered a job by the law firm
that was representing Searle. Later that same year, he resigned as
U.S. attorney and withdrew from the case, delaying the grand jury's
investigation. This caused the statute of limitations on the charges
to run out, and the investigation was dropped. *And* he accepted the
job with Searle's law firm.[24] Stunning.

In 1980, a review by the Public Board of Inquiry set up by the
FDA determined that aspartame should not be approved. The
board said it had "not been presented with proof of reasonable cer-
tainty that aspartame is safe for use as a food additive." In 1981, new
FDA Commissioner Arthur Hull Hayes was appointed. Despite the
fact that three out of six scientists advised against approval, Hayes

decided to overrule the scientific review panel and allow aspartame into limited dry goods. In 1983, he got it approved for beverages, even though the National Soft Drink Association urged the FDA to delay approval until further testing could be done. That same year, Hayes left the FDA amid charges of impropriety. The Internal Department of Health and Human Services was investigating Hayes for accepting gratuities from FDA-regulated companies. He went to work as a consultant for Searle's public relations firm. Interesting. The FDA finally urged Congress to prosecute Searle for giving the government false or incomplete test results on aspartame.[25] However, the two government attorneys assigned to the case decided not to prosecute. Later, they went to work for the law firm that represented Searle. Fascinating. Despite recognizing ninety-two different symptoms that result from ingesting aspartame, the FDA approved it for use, without restriction, in 1996.[26] Brilliant.

So many people have been sickened from this shit that there are aspartame victim support groups. Some of the ninety-two aspartame side effects listed by the FDA include memory loss, nerve cell damage, migraines, reproductive disorders, mental confusion, brain lesions, blindness, joint pain, Alzheimer's, bloating, nervous system disorders, hair loss, food cravings, and weight gain.[27]

Aspartame is a $1 billion industry.[28] The National Justice League has filed a series of lawsuits against food companies using aspartame, claiming they are poisoning the public. In September 2004, a class action lawsuit was filed for $350 million against NutraSweet and the American Diabetics Association. Secretary of Defense Donald Rumsfeld is named in the suit for using political muscle to get aspartame approved by the FDA.[29]

NutraSweet and Equal contain aspartame. When ingested, one of aspartame's ingredients, methyl alcohol, converts into formaldehyde, a deadly neurotoxin.[30] In addition to aspartame, Equal contains the amino acid phenylalanine. Phenylalanine occurs naturally in the brain. But high levels can increase the chance of seizures and lead to depression and schizophrenia.[31] There is no lesser of the two evils. NutraSweet and Equal are both evil. Sweet & Low is no saint, either. It is an artificial sweetener that contains saccharin, a coal-tar compound.[32] Stay away.

Because we're having so much fun, let's bash the shit out of Splenda, one of the newer sweeteners. Splenda is made by chlorinating sugar, changing its molecular structure. The finished product is called sucralose. The makers of this poison tout its lack of calories and claim it's safe for diabetics. The FDA calls sucralose 98 percent pure. The other 2 percent contains small amounts of heavy metals, methanol, and arsenic.[33] Well, gee, at least it doesn't have calories. So what if it has a little arsenic? Sucralose has been found to cause diarrhea; organ, genetic, immune system, and reproductive damage; swelling of the liver and kidneys; and a decrease in fetal body weight.[34] What a splendid product! According to Dr. Joseph Mercola in Consumer Research magazine's article "The Potential Dangers of Sucralose," "There is no clear-cut evidence that sugar substitutes are useful in weight reduction. On the contrary, there is some evidence that these substances may stimulate appetite."[35]

Not only have multiple class action lawsuits been filed, but even the president of the National Sugar Association and the manufacturer of Equal are up in arms about Splenda. They each filed suit, claiming that Splenda manufacturers are misleading consumers into thinking the product is natural when it is "a highly processed chemical compound." Don't think that the giants behind artificial sweeteners and the sugar industry suddenly started caring about public health. Splenda's clever marketing is just totally screwing up their sales. But even executive director for the Center for Science in the Public Interest, Dr. Michael F. Jacobson, who normally criticizes The National Sugar Association, had to agree: "Advertising and labeling, whether for products that are healthful or unhealthful, should be truthful and not misleading." [36]

Clearly, artificial sweeteners and refined sugars are bad for many reasons. Here's one more. We have a delicate balancing act occurring in our bodies at all times—pH balance. Basically, everything we eat has its own pH balance. When food is digested, it leaves an acid or alkaline "ash" in the body, depending on the food's mineral content. Surprise, surprise: Artificial sweeteners are highly acid forming. (Coffee, excessive protein, meat, pasteurized dairy, refined sugars, and fatty foods are, too.)[37]

When our bodies get too acidic, we are much more prone to illness. Sometimes, we don't even know we're sick until it's too late. But we can notice mild maladies, like skin problems, allergies, headaches, colds, or yeast infections. Or, we can experience major trauma—severe damage to our thyroid gland, liver, and adrenal glands. If our pH balance becomes too acidic, our bodies will react to protect themselves. To neutralize the acid, they will take alkalizing minerals from our reserves. If our reserves are low, the body will withdraw minerals from our bones and muscles.[38] If that doesn't scare you, consider this: It is commonly believed that cancer cells thrive in acid environments.[39]

Now, logically, you would think that citrus fruits are acidic, but actually, when they enter the body, they are alkalizing. We know this goes against the "use your own head" idea because they seem like they'd be acidic. But they contain potassium and calcium, which are alkalizing minerals. They also have a high percentage of alkaline salts. Nearly all fruits, vegetables, and legumes are alkaline when they enter the body.[40] Other alkalizing foods are sea vegetables, miso, soybeans, and tofu.

Fruit, good. Natural sweeteners, good. Refined sugars, bad. Artificial sweeteners, bad. Any questions?

Chapter 4

The Dead, Rotting, Decomposing Flesh Diet

The Atkins diet. Hmm. Eat the flesh of dead cows, dead pigs, and dead chickens. Avoid fresh fruit. You are a total moron if you think the Atkins diet will make you thin. Or, you are a gluttonous pig who wants to believe you can eat cheeseburgers all day long and lose weight. Perhaps you weren't listening the first time: You need to get healthy if you want to be skinny! Eating carcasses all day while avoiding fruit is a recipe for disaster. Of course, if you stop eating refined carbohydrates, you will lose weight. That's the part of the Atkins Diet that actually works. However, most of the weight you lose is water weight. You see, when our bodies metabolize protein (found in high amounts in meat and dairy), nitrogen waste is released in the form of urea. Urea is toxic and must be passed out of the body through urine. So the high-protein diet isn't ridding your body of fat. It's just serving as a diuretic—making you pee more to flush out the toxic urea.[41] But whether you lose this piss weight initially is inconsequential. You will be a fat, unhealthy, bloated pig if you live this way.

Trendy diets like Atkins become popular for one reason: They hide behind scientific jargon that *seems* to make sense and allow you to eat unhealthy, fattening foods as long as you avoid carbs. You believe in these diets because you want to. Most Americans eat twice as much protein as necessary, which has sent obesity, heart disease, and cancer rates soaring over the past fifty years. When you eat large amounts of animal protein and saturated fats and do not eat whole grains, vegetables, and fresh fruits, there is no fiber to bind all of the toxins and fat together to be eliminated from your body. You will eventually do an incredible amount of harm to yourself. Your poor kidneys are in serious jeopardy of developing stones, aging prematurely, and failing altogether. They must work twice as hard to break down protein and remove waste. By the time your blood shows the effects, it will be too late to reverse the damage. Diabetics are in even worse trouble with a high-protein diet because they are already at a higher risk of kidney disease to begin with. In a study involving 1,500 patients with diabetes, most had lost more than half of their kidney function because of a high intake of animal protein.[42] Don't care about your kidneys and just want to lose weight? The American Cancer Society conducted a study over a ten-year period with nearly 80,000 people trying to lose weight. Participants who ate meat three times a week or more gained substantially more weight than participants who avoided meat and consumed more vegetables.[43] Studies published in *The Journal of Clinical Nutrition and The New England Journal of Medicine* stated that meat eaters are much more likely to be overweight than vegetarians.[44]

Before you start spouting off information you've been brainwashed with about evolution and the food chain, read on. Yes, humans have a high level of intelligence. Yes, we created weapons for hunting and fire for cooking. Yes, we found a way to mass-produce animals for consumption. However, if you study animals in the wild, you will note that they do not rely on anything other than their natural hunting ability, speed, strength, claws, teeth, and jaws. They have no tools or weapons. Now look at yourself. Look at your flimsy fingernails in comparison to an eagle's talons. Look at your flat, blunt teeth compared to a lion's fangs. Compare your speed and agility to that of a tiger. Compare the strength of your jaw to a wolf's. Imagine yourself trying to run after an animal, catch it, and kill it using your bare hands, fingernails, teeth, and jaws. Not only would you look ridiculous, but you'd probably get your ass kicked, too. And even if you were successful, envision yourself eating the kill without the aid of an oven and silverware.[45] Yes, the human brain allows us to stay removed from the process of hunting. But does this mean we are "evolved" and "intelligent" and should be eating animal flesh just because we can? Man's "intelligence" also created alcohol, cigarettes, and drugs. Should we drink, smoke, and use just because we can?

Many meat eaters credit eating meat for our evolution from

cavemen into what we are now. Even if this were the case and eating meat did help us to evolve, look at what we evolved *from*. We looked liked friggin' apes and had massive heads, strong jaws, and brute strength. Maybe back then we were supposed to eat meat. But the last time we checked, we aren't cavemen anymore.

The second we put food in our mouths, the digestion process begins, thanks to our saliva. Guess what? Our alkaline saliva is not meant to break down animal flesh; carnivores have acid saliva, perfectly designed for the task. And hydrochloric acid, essential for digesting carcass, is secreted in very small amounts in our stomachs. However, the stomachs of carnivores have ten times more hydrochloric acid than ours. Our enzymes, digestive tracts, and organs are all different from those found in carnivores. Like it or not, our kidneys, colon, and liver are ill-equipped to process animal flesh. Compared to carnivores, our intestines are very long, so food that doesn't get adequately processed becomes clogged in our intestines. Animals quickly pass food through their digestive systems, but we have food rotting, decomposing, and fermenting in our intestinal tracts and colons, hence the need for colonics (aka: enemas). You don't see many tigers getting colonics, do you? You do see them napping, though. Even though their bodies are designed to digest meat, animals generally sleep all day while doing so because it is such a taxing process. Genetically and structurally, we are designed to thrive on plant foods.[46] Whether it is "lean meat" or a "skinless chicken breast," animal fat is still animal fat. Don't be fooled by terms coined by the meat industry. Your body can't handle animal fat, so it settles like lumpy shit all over your ass, thighs, sides, arms, and stomach.

And then there are the gross, stomach-turning realities of the meat-production industry.

Of the ten billion animals slaughtered each year in America for human consumption, the vast majority of them come from factory farms. Factory farms that raise cattle, pigs, chickens, egg-laying hens, veal calves, or dairy cows have an enormous amount of animals in a very small space. There are no vast meadows or lush, green pastures. The animals are confined inside buildings, where they are literally packed in on top of each other. Egg-laying hens are crammed into cages so small, they are unable to open their wings, and their mangled feet actually grow around the wire mesh floors. This overcrowded, stressful environment causes chickens to peck at each other and factory farm workers, so the ends of their beaks are seared off their faces using a hot knife. Pigs and cows are imprisoned in stalls so small, they are unable to turn around or lie down comfortably. Cattle are subject to third-degree branding burns and having their testicles and horns ripped out. Pigs also suffer from branding and castration, in addition to the mutilation of their ears, tails, and teeth. They all live in the filth of their own urine, feces, and vomit with infected, festering sores and wounds. To keep animals alive in these unsanitary conditions, farmers must give them regular doses of antibiotics.

Half of all the antibiotics made in the United States each year are administered to farm animals, causing antibiotic resistance in the humans who eat them.[47] A study at the University of California-Berkeley linked eating beef to urinary tract infections (UTIs) in women. It just so happens that the most common infectious disease in women is UTIs.[48] You do the math.

For shits and giggles, we've compiled a partial list of what's in meat, poultry, seafood, and dairy: benzene hexachloride (BHC), chlordane, dichlorodiphenyltrichloroethane (DDT), dieldrin, dioxin, heptachlor, hexachlorobenzene (HCB), and lindane.[49] Perhaps that's why eating "meat" has been linked to obesity; cancer; liver, kidney, lung, and reproductive disorders; birth defects; miscarriages; and nervous system disorders.[50] American farmers started using chemical pesticides in the late 1800s and were initially thrilled with the results. However, it was eventually noticed that pesticides were killing those who were most exposed to them: farmers, field workers, and animals. In 1972, the Environmental Protection Agency banned DDT.[51] But the pesticides that followed were even worse. BHC is 19 times more carcinogenic than DDT, chlordane 4 times more, dieldrin 47 to 85 times more, HCB 23 times more, and heptachlor 15 to 30 times more. By the late 1980s, of the 450 endangered animal species, more than half were threatened with extinction. The government finally called for a ban on the production and use of other pesticides. But this didn't stop these pesticides from reaching our food supply. Companies were allowed to use up their enormous stockpiles of these pesticides by selling them to countries outside of America. (Apparently, it was acceptable to poison people and animals as long as they weren't American.) These countries used the pesticides on their crops, which were then imported into the United States.[52] Brilliant, huh? And, banned or not, once they have entered the soil or water, pesticides can still poison for decades.[53]

One widely used herbicide, glufosinate, whose residues have been found in U.S. waters and food supplies, causes hormonal and brain damage.[54] In his book, *Diet for a Poisoned Planet,* David Steinman reports that of all the toxic chemicals found in food, 95 to 99 percent come from meat, fish, dairy, and eggs.[55] He also reveals that many of the tests performed don't even detect many chemicals and pesticides. The Food and Drug Administration's own Total Diet Study found that bacon had 48 different pesticide residues, bologna and other luncheon meats had 102 different industrial pollutants and pesticides, fast food hamburgers had 113 residues, hot dogs had 123, and ground beef had 82 industrial chemical and pesticide residues, just to name a few.[56] In comparison, meat contains 14 times more pesticides than plant foods, and dairy has 5 times more pesticides than plant foods. The United States alone uses *one billion pounds* of pesticides every year on our food. That, our pathetic contamination sampling process, and our use of growth hormones has caused the European Economic Community to reject our meat exportations on numerous occasions.[57]

Many animals are even given arsenic-laced drugs.[58] Arsenic!

Chemical pesticides are often sprayed directly onto the skin of animals to ward off parasites, insects, rodents, and fungi. In addition, these animals are given food treated with pesticides. On factory farms, bigger is better. More meat, milk, and eggs mean more money for the farmers. So to grow them larger or have them produce more, animals are given steroids and growth hormones. But what is happening to the people who eat these fattened animals? Young girls are experiencing an early onset of puberty at epidemic proportions. Many scientists attribute this to all of the hormones in chicken, meat, and milk that are forced upon children. Basically, every time you consume factory-farmed chicken, beef, veal, pork, eggs, or dairy, you are eating antibiotics, pesticides, steroids, and hormones. This is worth repeating: *Every time you consume factory-farmed chicken, beef, veal, pork, eggs, or dairy, you are eating antibiotics, pesticides, steroids, and hormones.*

Now you might be thinking, "Who cares about all this pesticide-cancer shit? I just want to get skinny!" Ever been on The Pill and gained weight? Ever gained weight from having fertility treatments? Well, eating animals that are given hormones has the same effect as if you were taking these directly. According to Dr. Paula

Baillie-Hamilton, author of *The Body Restoration Plan,* antibiotics alone can account for weight gain in animals.[59] She also states that the toxic chemicals used in food production are fattening. Whether it's the pesticides used for growing crops or the chemicals given to animals to fatten them up, they alter the body's metabolism in a way that causes weight gain. Having studied animals and humans, she discovered that low doses of toxic chemicals increased appetite, slowed metabolism, decreased ability to burn stored fat, and reduced ability to exercise.[60] The FDA lists approximately 1,700 drugs approved for use in animal feed. Of these approved drugs, approximately 300 include "weight gain" in their description.[61] However, in their book *Animal Factories,* Jim Mason and Peter Singer disclose an estimate of 20,000 to 30,000 different drugs actually being used.[62]

We constantly hear the snobby declaration, "I don't eat any red meat. I just eat chicken." Well now you know: Chicken is just as bad for you as cow or pig. In fact, it might even be worse. According to the American *Journal of Epidemiology,* eating chicken (and fish) is linked to colon cancer. Researchers examined the eating habits of 32,000 men and women over a six-year period and then monitored emerging cancer cases for the next six years. "Among participants who generally avoided red meat but who ate white meat less than once per week, colon cancer risk was 55 percent higher than for those who avoided both kinds of meat. Those who had white meat at least once per week had more than three-fold higher colon cancer risk." [63] Researchers at the National Cancer Institute found grilled chicken to have high levels of heterocyclic amines, carcinogens that are formed when animal proteins are heated. With 480 nanograms of heterocyclic amines per gram, grilled chicken registered 15 times higher than beef.[64]

Do not be lulled into a false sense of security that our government keeps food safe. News of the avian influenza epidemic came and went, but this disease is very real and can run rampant in poultry flocks. And according to a survey by the National Research Council, one chicken processing plant had 90 percent of its poultry contaminated with salmonellosis.[65] Ninety fucking percent! Nasty.

Unfortunately, our waters aren't any better than our land. Yes, some fish contain essential fatty acids and vitamins, minerals, and protein. But you can easily get all these nutrients from flaxseeds; pumpkin, sesame, and sunflower seeds; nuts; soybeans; fruits; vegetables; leafy greens; soy products; and whole grains. Fish and other seafood contain high levels of contaminants from industrial and environmental pollutants, waste products, and pesticide residues from farms. Also present in fish and seafood are high levels of mercury and PCBs, which are well absorbed by the body. Other notables are BHC, chlordane, DDT, dieldrin, heptachlor, and dioxin.[66] These chemicals can cause neurotoxicity, which impairs a person's mental state and ability. The human body contains acetylcholine, a naturally occurring chemical that helps impulses pass from nerve to nerve. Once the impulse is passed, the chemical is no longer needed and is actually harmful if it remains. So our bodies produce an enzyme, cholinesterase, which rids us of the unwanted acetylcholine. Pesticides inhibit our ability to produce cholinesterase, which causes a buildup of the now-dangerous acetylcholine.[67] Mercury, a suspected carcinogen, can alter immune function, raise blood pressure, cause blindness or paralysis, increase the chance of cardiac mortality, and is known to reduce fertility and virility.[68] It can also inflict permanent brain damage on fetuses, infants, and children.

Appetizing, huh? Have some mercury poisoning with your ahi tuna. How about some trichinosis with your pork? Don't forget a side of salmonella with your eggs or chicken. We certainly don't want to leave out an order of mad cow disease. Think about what you've been eating. What we call salmon, hamburger, steak, chicken, bacon, sausage, ham, roast beef, salami, bologna, turkey, hot dog, and duck are actually decomposing, rotting animal carcasses. *Bon appétit!*

Closing your eyes to the problem will not make it go away. You don't want to see it, but you'll *eat* it? So, yeah, if you want to get skinny, you've got to be a vegetarian—someone who doesn't eat dead animals or seafood. Quit whining. We weren't raised by hippie-crunchy-granola parents on vegetarian communes. Growing up, we both ate meat all day, every day. We scoffed at tofu and spit on vegetables. Really. Kim's addictions included such delicacies as corned beef hash, canned Vienna sausages, and daily Big Macs. Every single day in 1992, Rory ate a ham, egg, and cheese sandwich for breakfast, followed by a bacon double cheeseburger, fries, and a soda for lunch. Dinner was always a dead chicken, fish, cow, or pig. Now granted, we didn't give up meat just to get skinny. We both became vegetarians after learning about the treatment of farm animals. But we each noticed big changes in our minds, attitudes, health, moods, and asses when we gave up carcass. So before you say, "I could never give up meat," realize that nearly every single vegetarian on the planet said those same words. Then shut the fuck up, look at an inspirational picture of a skinny bitch, and clean out your freezer.

There are a ton of awesome, soy-based fake meat products on the market. Not only do they taste great, but soy has been lauded for lowering cholesterol, protecting against cancer, reducing the risk of heart attacks,[69] and helping the body to better utilize calcium. Phytoestrogens, found in soy, help protect women from breast cancer and can alleviate menopausal symptoms.[70] However, there are opponents to soy, who claim that it can negatively impact the thyroid, cause mineral deficiencies, and raise the risk of breast cancer. But according to health expert Dr. Andrew Weil, "There is still much to be learned about soy, but the majority of research so far has shown that it's a safe and nutritious food when eaten in reasonable amounts—about one or two daily servings."[71] We encourage you to think for yourself and make your own decision.

If you decide to eat soy products that imitate meat products, know that these foods may not taste exactly like the real thing. But once you get rid of your meat addiction, you'll be satisfied with the substitutes. You just need to spend a few weeks (and dollars) experimenting until you find the ones you like. Veggie burgers exist by the dozen. Health Is Wealth makes fake buffalo wings that taste so good, your pubes will fall out. Gardenburger's Flame-Grilled Chik'n is so amazing, you might have to kill yourself. Lightlife has a kick-ass line of "cold cuts" and fabulous "bacon." One amazing website is *www.vegieworld.com*. It is an Asian mail order company that not only sells fake chicken and meat, but has fake seafood, too. But you don't have to look far: Seek and ye shall find. We list lots of meatless wonders in Chapter 11. But remember, getting skinny means using your head. You must read all the ingredients and make sure there are *no* animal products in anything you buy. For the rest of your skinny life, every time you buy something that you will be swallowing, you must read the ingredients.

Chapter 5

The Dairy Disaster

G o suck your mother's tits. Go on. Suck your mother's tits. You think this is ridiculous? It is. Get ready to use your head.

When a woman gives birth, her body produces milk and she nurses her child.

Breast milk can grow an 8-pound newborn into a 24-pound toddler. Sounds pretty fattening, huh? It is. By design, it is intended to allow for the biggest growth spurt of a person's entire life. Breast milk alone can accommodate for a 300 percent weight gain in a twelve-month period. When her child is anywhere from 12 to 24 months old, a mother stops breast feeding. Her milk dries up. The child will never drink breast milk ever again.

Cows, like all mammals, are much the same. Their bodies produce milk only when they give birth. Contrary to popular belief, they do not need to be milked—ever. Their udders, like women's breasts, exist even when there is no milk in them. There is one major difference, however. Cows' milk, by design, grows a 90-pound calf into a 2,000-pound cow over the course of two years.[72] It allows calves to double their birth weight in forty-seven days and leaves their four stomachs feeling full. Sounds even more fattening than human milk, right? It is. It should be. Cows are bigger than humans. And the inner workings of their bodies are completely different than ours, which they should be. They are cows. We are humans. Duh.

Mammals need the enzyme lactase to digest lactose (the sugar found in dairy). However, between the ages of 18 months and 4 years, we lose 90 to 95 percent of this enzyme. The undigested lactose and the acidic nature of pasteurized milk encourage the growth of bacteria in our intestines.[73] All this contributes to a greater risk of cancer because cancer cells thrive in acidic conditions.[74]

Got mucus? Dairy products produce mucus, and often, the body will develop a cold or "allergies" to fight the dairy invasion.[75] Mother Nature is no fool. All species, including ours, have just what we need to get by. She did not intend for grownups to suck their mothers' tits. We don't need our mothers' milk as adults, just like grown cows don't need their mothers' milk anymore. We are the only species on the planet that drinks milk as adults. We are also the only species on the planet that drinks the milk of another species. We could be putting gorilla milk on our cereal or having zebra milk and cookies. Why cows' milk? Using the animal that produces the largest quantity of milk but is more easily housed than an elephant means more money for farmers. It has nothing to do with health or nutrition. Again, it all comes back to money. The dairy industry is a multibillion-dollar industry based on brilliant marketing and the addictive taste of milk, butter, and cheese. It has convinced most doctors, consumers, and government agencies that we *need* cows' milk. We have been told our whole lives, "You need milk to grow. Without milk, your bones will break. If you don't drink milk, you'll get osteoporosis. You need the calcium." *Bullshit*.

Researchers at Harvard, Yale, Penn State, and the National Institutes of Health have studied the effects of dairy intake on bones.
Not one of these studies found dairy to be a deterrent to osteoporosis.[76] On the contrary, a study funded by the National Dairy Council
itself revealed that the high protein content of dairy actually leaches
calcium from the body.[77] After looking at thirty-four published studies in sixteen countries, researchers at Yale University found that
the countries with the highest rates of osteoporosis—including the
United States, Sweden, and Finland—were those in which people
consumed the most meat, milk, and other animal foods.[78] Another
study showed that though 40 million American women have osteoporosis, only 250,000 African women have bone disease. In fact, of
the forty tribes in Kenya and Tanzania, only one—the Maasai—has
members suffering from osteoporosis. The Maasai, as it happens,
are a cattle-owning, milk-drinking tribe.[79]

Dairy products have been linked to a host of other problems,
too, including acne, anemia, anxiety, arthritis, attention deficit disorder, attention deficit hyperactivity disorder, fibromyalgia,
headaches, heartburn, indigestion, irritable bowel syndrome, joint
pain, osteoporosis, poor immune function,[80] allergies, ear infec-

tions, colic, obesity, heart disease, diabetes, autism, Crohn's disease, breast and prostate cancers,[81] and ovarian cancer.[82]

Harvey and Marilyn Diamond, authors of best-selling follow-up *Fit For Life II,* clearly state, "DAIRY PRODUCTS ARE DISEASE-PRODUCING. They're harmful. They *cause* suffering. They're the perfect thing to eat if you want to be sick and have a diseased body. The dietitians and nutritionists who are mouthpieces and cheerleaders for the dairy industry, telling you that dairy products are a good food, should hide their heads in shame—not only for leading the innocent to believe that dairy products are actually valuable, but also for failing to keep abreast of the field about which they are *supposed* to know something."

Yes, we are saying it is common knowledge in the medical research field that dairy is bad for you. Yes, we are saying that executives in the dairy industry are well aware of this fact but make claims that milk "does a body good." How do they get away with this? Easily. They spend hundreds of millions of dollars every year to market their products. And average consumers don't spend their time perusing medical journals, but they do read magazines and watch television.

What about medical doctors? Why do they believe that milk is beneficial? It is a sad fact that in this country, most doctors know almost nothing about nutrition. According to a Senate investigation, doctors receive *less than three hours* of nutritional training in medical school.[83] They have been duped like the rest of us.

Let's pretend for a moment that cows' milk is healthy for humans. Even if it were, by the time factory farms were done with it, it wouldn't be. Dioxin, one of the most toxic substances in the world, is often found in dairy products.[84] And remember, for factory farms, higher production means bigger profits. When you consume dairy products, you are ingesting the same antibiotics, pesticides, steroids, and hormones you would if you ate meat directly. Cows are injected with bovine growth hormone. Their udders, under normal conditions, would supply about ten pounds of milk a day. Greedy farmers have their cows producing up to a hundred pounds of milk a day! There is no gentle farmer milking the cow with a bucket between his feet. Cows are milked by machine; metal clamps are attached to the cows' sensitive udders. The udders become sore and infected. Pus forms. But the machines keep on milking, sucking the dead white blood cells into the milk.[85] How freaking gross is that? To get rid of all the bacteria and other shit, milk must be pasteurized. But pasteurization destroys beneficial enzymes and makes calcium less available without even killing all the viruses or bacteria. Hell, even radioactive particles are found in milk![86]

But don't the government and U.S. Department of Agriculture protect us from all this? Hell no. Sickeningly high levels of pesticides found in dairy meet government standards. Records from the Food and Drug Administration show that "virtually 100% of the cheese products produced and sold in the U.S. has detectable pesticide residues." [87]

Milk is not a reliable source of minerals. You get much higher levels of manganese, chromium, selenium, and magnesium from fruits and vegetables. Fruits and veggies are also high in boron, which helps lessen the loss of calcium through urine.[88] Consuming high amounts of dairy blocks iron absorption, contributing to iron deficiency.[89]

So do you need calcium by the trough? Nope. A simple way to get adequate calcium is by including the following foods in your diet: fortified grains, kale, collard greens, mustard greens, cabbage, kelp, seaweed, watercress, chickpeas, broccoli, red beans, soybeans, tofu, seeds (sesame seeds rate among the highest), and raw nuts. It is just that simple. But don't be looking to pop a calcium pill as a quick fix. Research shows that supplements do not make a significant difference in preventing or treating osteoporosis.[90] Good news: Fifteen minutes of direct sunlight every day aides in Vitamin D absorption, which means stronger bones.

How about eggs, you ask? When a woman is pregnant and she drinks alcohol or does drugs, it affects her unborn child, right? Right. Well, it is the same with chickens and their unhatched eggs. When you eat eggs, you are ingesting all the same hormones, pesticides, chemicals, and steroids as if you were eating the chicken directly. So if you really believe that eating "just egg whites" isn't fattening, we've got a bridge we can sell ya. Eggs are high in saturated fat and are completely disgusting when you think about what you are eating. Try that for once. Actually think about what you are eating!

You will pee in your pants when you see how much weight you lose from giving up dairy. The fat in cheese is what gives it the taste and texture we love. Of the calories found in cheese, 70 to 80 percent come from fat. Even if you're buying the low-fat, part-skim nonsense, more than half the calories come from fat.[91] Fat free?

Give us a freaking break! Remember what milk is for. It is designed to fatten up baby cows. Do you really believe it can be made fat free? Get your head out of your ass. Milk = fat. Butter = fat. Cheese = fat. People who think these products can be low fat or fat free = fucking morons.

Luckily, there are many alternatives to dairy products. Not only do grocery stores carry these items, but many coffee shops now offer soymilk and some bakeries are selling dairy-free desserts. A personal favorite-tasting milk substitute is Rice Dream (Original Enriched), which is fortified with vitamins and calcium. But feel free to experiment until you find your own favorite brand. Remember to read the ingredients. Avoid the milk substitutes that contain sugar. Instead of butter, try Earth Balance Natural Buttery Spread or Soy Garden Natural Buttery Spread, both made from nonhydrogenated oils. Can't live without ice cream? You don't have to. Soy Delicious has incredible knock-offs, which are completely dairy free. They even make must-have flavors, such as Chunky Mint Madness, Cookie Avalanche, Rocky Road, and Peanut Butter Zigzag. They also have a line of "ice creams" and sorbets that are fruit-sweetened! Dairy and sugar free! Too exciting for words! We're also huge fans of Double Rainbow Soy Cream, another amazing ice cream alternative. Are you a cheese addict? No problem. Follow Your Heart's Vegan Gourmet makes a kick-ass substitute in mozzarella, Monterey jack, and nacho. It even melts! It rules. Beware of the many brands that tout themselves as "soy cheese," leading consumers to believe they're dairy free. When you get past the misleading packaging and actually read the ingredients, you'll discover sneaky dairy ingredients like whey or casein. Steer clear. Other brands are completely dairy-free, but they taste like shit.

Need eggs in your life? Easy peasy. Egg Beaters are made of real eggs, so they're a gross no-no. But if you pan-fry House Tofu Steak (slice it in half first) and add a little soy butter, salt, pepper, and ketchup, you've got yourself a fried "egg." There's also an egg substitute in powder form for cooking and baking called Ener-G egg replacer. And many markets sell a pretty good tofu "egg" salad.

As the demand grows for healthy, yummy, animal-free, dairy-free products, more companies will supply us with these foods. So let your consumer dollars voice your desire, and your body will be rewarded. And don't be shy. If your grocery store doesn't carry something you want, open your fat mouth and ask for it.

Chapter 6

You Are What You Eat

N ow would be a good time to reflect on the old adage, "You are what you eat." This statement, in all its simplicity, is brilliant. You are what you eat. You are a human body comprised of organs, blood and guts, and other shit. The food you put into your body works its way through your organs and bloodstream and is actually part of who you are. So every time you put crap in your body, you are crap.

If Chapters 4 and 5 didn't convince you to avoid eating animal products (crap), maybe this will. Even knowing how abysmal the living conditions are for animals on factory farms, you cannot begin to imagine what the slaughter practices are like. "Humane" protocol calls for animals to be "stunned" before they are slaughtered. For cows, this means getting a metal bolt shot into the skull and then retracted. When done properly, using working equipment, this renders the cow unconscious. But time is money, and slaughterhouses operate at lightning speeds, some killing one animal every three seconds. Because thousands of frightened, struggling cows are not easy to stun, it is extremely common for a "stunner" to miss his mark.[92] Panicked hogs, also difficult to "hit," are stunned with an electric device. And if the jolt is too high, it bruises and bloodies the hogs' flesh (bad for business). Because business comes first on factory farms, the jolt is lowered, despite the fact that it doesn't properly stun the hogs.[93]

Stunned or not, cows and hogs are then "strung up" from the ceiling by a chain attached to their leg(s).[94] In theory, while they dangle there, they are supposed to be unconscious. But often they are fully conscious, struggling, screaming, and fearfully staring at the workers while they have their throats stabbed open.[95] Next, they travel along a "bleed rail," where they should bleed to death. But again, these large, frightened, struggling, conscious animals are difficult targets and the "stickers" (workers who cut their throats) don't always get a "good cut." Before cows can bleed to death, they are sent on their way to the "head-skinners," where the skin is sliced from their heads while they are still conscious.[96] Of course, this is excruciatingly painful, and the cows kick and struggle frantically. To avoid getting injured by the struggling animal, workers will sometimes sever the spinal cord with a knife blow to the back of the head. This paralyzes the animal below the neck so that the worker is safe. But these cows can still feel their skin being sliced away from their faces.[97] Next, their legs and head are chopped off, their entrails removed from their bodies, and then, finally, they are split in half. Often before hogs can bleed to death, they are dunked fully conscious into 140-degree scalding water to remove the hair from their bodies.[98]

Chickens, because they are so overcrowded and stressed, frequently peck each other and factory farm workers, so the ends of their beaks are literally chopped off their faces. Even though they currently comprise more than 95 percent of all animals slaughtered for food, Congress exempted chickens (and turkeys) from the Humane Slaughter Act, so there is no requirement to stun them[99] (not that it would matter, anyway). But because it is easier to handle chickens that aren't fighting for their lives, their heads are sometimes dragged through a water bath that has been electrically charged. This paralyzes the birds, but does not render them unconscious.[100] They are snatched up, shackled upside down, and their throats are slashed by machine at the rate of thousands per hour.[101] Next, they are dunked in scalding water to loosen their feathers. Again, they are supposed to be dead at this point, but if the machine misses its mark, or the chickens haven't bled to death, they are "boiled" alive. Then they are placed into a series of machines that literally beat their feathers off of them, still alive and having just been scalded.[102] All the while, they are being handled like rubber toys: grabbed by their necks, feet, or wings and thrown around. You get the idea.

In egg-laying factories, male baby chicks are completely useless to farmers because they don't produce eggs. So workers snatch up chicks speeding by on a conveyer belt, quickly glance at their undersides, and then toss the "useless" males into the garbage. Yes. Literally. Millions of male baby chicks are piled on top of each other in garbage dumpsters—left to die.

In her book, *Slaughterhouse,* Gail Eisnitz, chief investigator for the Humane Farming Association, interviewed dozens of slaughter-house workers throughout the country. *Every single one* admitted to abusing animals or neglecting to report those who did.[103] The following are quotes from slaughterhouse workers taken from her book. (They are quite graphic and difficult to read, but we implore you to read each one. It is important to know what our dietary desires are contributing to. Surely you can endure reading it if animals have to endure suffering it):

"I seen them take those stunners—they're about as long as a yard stick—and shove it up the hog's ass. . . They do it with cows, too. . . And in their ears, their eyes, down their throat. . . They'll be squealing and they'll just shove it right down there."[104]

"Hogs get stressed out pretty easy. If you prod them too much they have heart attacks. If you get a hog in a chute that's had the shit prodded out of him and has a heart attack or refuses to move, you take a meat hook and hook it into his bunghole [anus]. You're dragging these hogs alive, and a lot of times the meat hook rips out of the bunghole. I've seen hams—thighs—completely ripped open. I've also seen intestines come out. If the hog collapses near the front of the chute, you shove the meat hook into his cheek and drag him forward."[105]

"Or in their mouth. The roof of their mouth. And they're still alive."[106]

"Pigs on the kill floor have come up and nuzzled me like a puppy. Two minutes later I had to kill them—beat them to death with a pipe."[107]

"These hogs get up to the scalding tank, hit the water and start screaming and kicking. Sometimes they thrash so much they kick water out of the tank. . . . Sooner or later they drown. There's a rotating arm that pushes them under, no chance for them to get out. I'm not sure if they burn to death before they drown, but it takes them a couple of minutes to stop thrashing."[108]

"Sometimes I grab it [a hog] by the ear and stick it right through the eye. I'm not just taking its eye out, I'll go all the way to the hilt, right up through the brain, and wiggle the knife."[109]

"Only you don't just kill it, you go in hard, push hard, blow the windpipe, make it drown in its own blood. Split its nose. A live hog would be running around the pit. It would just be looking up at me and I'd be sticking, and I would just take my knife and—cut its eye out while it was just sitting there. And this hog would just scream."[110]

"I could tell you horror stories . . . about cattle getting their heads stuck under the gate guards, and the only way you can get it out is to cut their heads off while they're still alive."[111]

"He'll kick them [hogs], fork them, use anything he can get his hands on. He's already broken three pitchforks so far this year, just jabbing them. He doesn't care if he hits its eyes, head, butt. He jabs them so hard he busts the wooden handles. And he clubs them over the back."[112]

"I've seen live animals shackled, hoisted, stuck, and skinned. Too many to count, too many to remember. It's just a process that's continually there. I've seen shackled beef looking around before they've been stuck. I've seen hogs [that are supposed to be lying down] on the bleeding conveyor get up after they've been stuck. I've seen hogs in the scalding tub trying to swim."[113]

"I seen guys take broomsticks and stick it up the cow's behind, screwing them with a broom."[114]

"I've drug cows till their bones start breaking, while they were still alive. Bringing them around the corner and they get stuck up in the doorway, just pull them till their hide be ripped, till the blood just drip on the steel and concrete. Breaking their legs. . . . And the cow be crying with its tongue stuck out. They pull him till his neck just pop."[115]

"One time I took my knife—it's sharp enough—and I sliced off the end of a hog's nose, just like a piece of bologna. The hog went crazy for a few seconds. Then it just sat there looking kind of stupid. So I took a handful of salt brine and ground it into his nose. Now that hog really went nuts, pushing its nose all over the place. I still had a bunch of salt left in my hand—I was wearing a rubber glove—and I stuck the salt right up the hog's ass. The poor hog didn't know whether to shit or go blind."[116]

"Nobody knows who's responsible for correcting animal abuse at the plant. The USDA does zilch."[117]

Eisnitz chronicled the constant failure of U.S. Department of Agriculture inspectors to stop this abuse and their willingness to look the other way. In addition, she exposed the USDA's blatant tolerance for allowing contaminated meat into the human food supply. Think about it. *Ten billion* animals a year! Do you think the USDA has enough inspectors to supervise the humane and safe slaughter of *10 billion* animals a year? Of course the inspectors tolerate abuse and contaminated meat. Imagine the kind of person who would have a job that entailed witnessing the slaughter of thousands of innocent animals every day. Even if every single inspector did a good job (they don't), the factory workers can easily bypass the system. Eisnitz interviewed one worker from a horse slaughterhouse, who said, "Might be part of him's [a contaminated horse] bad, might be the pneumonia's traveled everywhere. I'd drag him back, and my boss would tell me to cut the hindquarters off and bring him into the cooler. The meat's supposed to be condemned, but still you'd cut it up and bag it." When Eisnitz asked, "But don't they have to be stamped 'USDA inspected?' " he responded, "He [his boss] got the stamper. He can stamp it himself when the doc leaves. . . . You take a condemned horse, skin him, cut him up, sell the meat. . . . We've sold it as beef."[118]

According to the Congressional testimony of one former Perdue worker, the poultry plants are filthy. She said there were flies, rats, and 5-inch long flying cockroaches covering the walls and floors.[119] Believe it or not, it gets worse: "After they are hung, sometimes the chickens fall off into the drain that runs down the middle of the line. This is where roaches, intestines, diseased parts, fecal contamination, and blood are washed down. Workers [vomit] into the drain. . . . Employees are constantly chewing and spitting out snuff and tobacco on the floor . . . sometimes they have to relieve themselves on the floor. . . . The Perdue supervisors told us to take the fallen chickens out of the drain and send them down the line."[120] A USDA inspector said of the cockroaches, "One time we shined a flashlight into a hole they were crawling in and out, and they were so thick it was like maggots, you couldn't even see the surface."[121] A worker at another poultry plant said, "Every day, I saw black chicken, green chicken, chicken that stank, and chicken with feces on it. Chicken like this is supposed to be thrown away, but instead it would be sent down the line to be processed."[122] Another worker at another plant said, "I personally have seen rotten meat—you can tell by the odor. This rotten meat is mixed with the fresh meat and sold for baby food. We are asked to mix it with the fresh food, and this is the way it is sold. You can see the worms inside the meat."[123] No comment. We are simply speechless.

Animals are intelligent, emotional, social creatures. Researchers at Bristol University in Britain discovered that cows actually nurture friendships and bear grudges. One study showed cows displaying excitement while solving intellectual challenges.[124]

Chickens are as smart as mammals, including some primates,

claims animal behaviorist Dr. Chris Evans of Macquarie University in Australia. They are apt pupils and can learn by watching the mistakes of others. One researcher conducted a study that demonstrated chickens' ability to use switches and levers to change the temperature of their surroundings. A PBS documentary revealed chickens' love for television and music.[125]

Pigs can play video games! They've been labeled as more intelligent than dogs and three-year-old humans. They too can indicate their temperature preferences.[126]

Even fish have feelings. Dr. Donald Broom, scientific adviser to the British government, explains, "The scientific literature is quite clear. Anatomically, physiologically and biologically, the pain system in fish is virtually the same as in birds and animals." Fish, like "higher vertebrates," have neurotransmitters similar to endorphins that relieve suffering. Of course, the only reason for their nervous systems to produce painkillers is to relieve pain.[127]

Animals hear the screaming and crying of other animals being slaughtered and are terrified. They know they are about to be killed and they are panic-stricken. When their young are taken from them, cows kick stall walls in rage and frustration and literally cry with grief.

Think of how you feel when you are angry, afraid, and grief-stricken. Bear in mind the physical feelings that accompany these emotions. These emotions—fear, grief, and rage—produce chemical changes in our bodies. They do the same to animals. Their blood pressures rise. Adrenaline courses through their bodies. You are eating high blood pressure, stress, and adrenaline. You are eating fear, grief, and rage. You are eating suffering, horror, and murder. You are eating cruelty. You are what you eat. You cannot be thin and beautiful with a glowing complexion when you eat fear, grief, and rage.

Although a minuscule percentage of "meat" in the United States comes from free-range farms, how do you even know it is really free-range? Companies want us to believe that products labeled "free-range" or "free-roaming" are derived from animals that spent their short lives outdoors, enjoying sunshine, fresh air, and the company of other animals. But labels—other than "organic" on egg cartons—are not subject to any government regulations. In addition, the USDA doesn't regulate "free-range" or "free-roaming" claims for beef products.[128] Because there are no agencies governing these claims, do you take the word of someone who makes a living on blood money? And even if the farm was free-range and humane, the animals are still being sent to horrific slaughterhouses. (An undercover video of a kosher slaughterhouse revealed animals suffering the same abuse and torture.)[129] Many animals don't even survive the transport from their factory or free-range farm to slaughter. The only law in existence dictating care for transported animals is related to *train* transport. But it just so happens that 95 percent of animals are transported by *truck*.[130] They receive no food or water and no protection from the elements. Hundreds of thousands of animals are dead on arrival or too injured or sick to move. They don't get to stop for bathroom breaks, so the animals are forced to stand in their own urine and feces. In the wintertime, the animals' flesh and feet will actually freeze to the bottom and sides of the truck. So upon arrival, they are literally ripped away from the truck. One worker interviewed by Eisnitz said, "They freeze to that steel railing. They're still alive, and they'll hook a cable on it and pull it out, maybe pull a leg off."[131]

Assuming you started with a healthy animal (highly unlikely), you've now eaten hormones, pesticides, steroids, antibiotics, fear, grief, and rage. You are what you eat. But what if the animal wasn't healthy? Animals that are too sick or injured to walk are literally dragged to slaughter, one end of a chain attached to the animal, the other to a truck. The USDA still allowed these animals, referred to as "downers," to be slaughtered for human consumption until 2004. Finally, with the outbreak of more mad cow disease cases (a deadly and incurable disease that can be transmitted to humans through the consumption of cow flesh), they came to their senses. But in 2005, USDA Secretary Mike Johanns announced that downed animals may once again be slaughtered for human food. So in addition to all the other filth you're eating, you're also eating whatever illness the animal had. You are what you eat.

Let's make believe that all the animals killed for human consumption are healthy, happy, free of antibiotics, steroids, and pesticides and are humanely raised and slaughtered. Pretend you are eating "perfect meat." Great. But what exactly are you eating? "Meat" is the decomposing, decaying, rotting flesh of a dead animal. As soon as an animal dies, it starts "breaking down." How long has passed between when the animal was slaughtered and the time you are eating it? It could be weeks, even months. You want to put a dead animal corpse—that has been rotting away for months— in your mouth? In your body? Because meat is muscle tissue, it oxidizes in an open environment and turns brown. So most meat markets will scrape off the brown parts to make it look more appealing. Another trick of the trade is using tinted lighting in open meat cases to enhance the meat's color.[132] Restaurants and ranchers might call their meat "aged to perfection," but no matter how you slice it, it's still a putrefying corpse. You are what you eat.

Just because you can't see what's happening doesn't mean it doesn't exist. Every time you have a craving for meat or dairy, remember what goes on inside every slaughterhouse, processing plant, and grocery store. Linda McCartney said it best: "If slaughterhouses had glass walls, we'd all be vegetarians."[133] For added motivation with your new lifestyle, visit GoVeg.com and order a free vegetarian starter kit.

So now you are officially vegan, a person who doesn't eat *any* animal products. No meat, chicken, pork, fish, eggs, milk, cheese, or butter. Feel great about it. Yes, it is challenging to avoid these foods, but you will reap the karmic rewards of being vegan (like being skinny). For starters, you're sparing the lives of at least ninety animals a year.[134] And every environmentalist knows that factory farming is completely destroying the environment. As ridiculous as it sounds, the methane resulting from the burps and farts of 10 billion animals a year is directly responsible for global warming.[135] The urine and feces are polluting and contaminating soil and water all over the country. According to the Environmental Protection Agency, they are the largest polluters of U.S. waterways.[136] Moreover, the amount of land, food, water, and energy used to raise 10 billion animals a year for slaughter could be used to grow food for *all of the starving people in the world.* That's right—you being vegan is actually a step toward ending world hunger. Now that's some serious skinny karma.

So you shouldn't eat cows, chickens, pigs, fish, milk, cheese, or eggs. So what the hell should you eat? Pretty much everything else: fruits, vegetables, legumes, nuts, seeds, and whole grains. Deep down, you've known all along that these foods are best for you; now it's time to get back on track. Our diets have strayed so far off course from where they belong; we've allowed meat to take center stage, with grains and vegetables playing supporting roles. Wrong, wrong, wrong. There is a plethora of great-tasting, healthy, wholesome foods that you've likely been neglecting for years. Well, those days are over.

Can you remember back to your grade-school days when you

learned about photosynthesis? Plants store the sun's energy, which we receive by eating them. If you can, just picture the light energy from the sun beaming down to the vegetables and fruits, and as we eat those foods, imagine that energy being transmitted into our bodies. Our nervous systems are maintained and stimulated by this light. What an amazing gift from nature—to be able to eat such pure foods that give our bodies so much!

However, be advised, all fruits and vegetables are not created equal. Plants need vitamins and minerals to function and grow properly. When they are sprayed with pesticides and grown in chemically treated soil, they won't absorb all the proper nutrients. This results in a loss of enzymes. So, organic fruits and vegetables—ones that have been grown in pure, untreated soil and without pesticides—have far more enzymes than their conventionally grown counterparts.[137]

Any scientist can tell you that food has an "energy" or "life" to it. Anyone with common sense can tell you that eating a live, fresh fruit is healthier than eating a cooked, canned, preserved one. Why? Because this "life" comes from the plant's energy, nutrients, phytochemicals, and enzymes. Enzymes are living biochemical factors that we need to survive. They are critical for digestion, breathing, reproduction, and the functioning of DNA and RNA. They also help repair and heal our organs, detoxify our bodies, carry out our nerve impulses, and help us think.

There are three types of enzymes: metabolic, digestive, and food enzymes. Fortunately, we produce our own metabolic enzymes, which run the whole body, maintain our health, and defend us from illness and infection. But our own enzyme supplies are limited. So to continue healthy bodily functions, we need to supplement with food. When we eat, our bodies release digestive enzymes to break down the food. If we eat foods devoid of enzymes, such as meat, processed food, and even just overcooked food (high temperatures destroy enzymes), our bodies have to work much harder.[138] Harder work means using more of our precious enzymes. Over time, this can result in an enlargement of the digestive organs and the endocrine glands. (Studies have shown that the increased weight of these organs accompanies obesity.)[139] This lack of enzymes can also cause a disruption in the body's ability to make enough metabolic enzymes. But when we eat foods high in enzymes, such as fruits, salad, or lightly steamed veggies, we get an enzyme boost along with the meal, so our bodies don't have to work so hard. There is no greater defender of our bodies than enzymes. When not in use for digestion, enzymes are busy repairing and cleaning our bodies.[140] So don't go throwing your enzymes away on shit!

So how do we get these enzymes into our bodies? We just need to make the following foods part of our daily diets: fruits (especially pineapples, papayas, bananas, and mangos), raw or lightly steamed vegetables, raw nuts and seeds, wheat grass, sea vegetables, garlic, and legumes. Juicing is a great way to detoxify your body and get a lot of enzymes, but you must drink it right away.[141] As soon as a fruit is peeled, or cut, or juiced, it begins to lose its enzymes.[142] So, buying a gallon of fresh-squeezed juice isn't as beneficial as making your own daily. Packaged juice has been pasteurized, and the heat destroys the enzymes. Granted, it's still better to drink pasteurized juice than soda. So if you can't juice for yourself, do the best you can.

Well, there you have it. Fruits and vegetables are the answer. And unless you are an idiot who wants cancer, obesity, and enlarged organs, organic is the way to go. You are what you eat.

Chapter 7

The Myths and Lies About Protein

If we had a penny for every time some meathead asked us, "So where do you get your protein?" we'd be richer than Oprah. Have you ever, ever, ever, in your entire life, heard of anyone suffering from a protein deficiency? Did you ever see an elephant, moose, or giraffe jonesing for a protein fix? If you weren't blacked out on bourbon for the past three chapters, you should know by now: It is a complete myth that we need a massive amount of protein. Too much protein—especially animal protein—can impair our kidneys; leach calcium, zinc, vitamin B, iron, and magnesium from our bodies; and cause osteoporosis, heart disease, cancer, and obesity. In addition, high amounts of protein can damage our tissues, organs, and cells, contributing to faster aging.[143] Yikes! Know this: People in other cultures consume half the amount of protein that we do, yet they live longer, healthier lives.[144]

Although too much is harmful, protein is still vital to our health. Protein produces enzymes, hormones, neurotransmitters, and antibodies; replaces worn out cells; transports various substances throughout the body; and aids in growth and repair.[145]

So how much protein do we really need? Well, depending who you ask, that number varies anywhere from 18 to 60 grams a day. But one thing is certain: Vegetarians need not worry. Researchers at Harvard found that vegetarians (who don't live on junk food) get adequate amounts of protein in their diets.[146] The American Dietetic Association reports that eating a vegetarian diet provides twice the amount of protein needed daily.[147] In his book, *Optimal Health,* Dr. Patrick Holford explains that "most people are in more

danger of eating too much protein than too little."[148] So pick something else to be neurotic about.

How do vegans get protein? Simply. We eat lentils, beans, nuts,
seeds, fruits, vegetables, whole grains, and soy products (edamame,
tofu, imitation cheeses and meats). When you eat well-balanced
meals consisting of these foods, you are guaranteed to get sufficient
protein. For example, for lunch, if you had a soy burger on a whole
grain bun with avocado and tomato and a small side salad, you'd get
22 grams of protein. See how easy? If you want an extra boost, treat
yourself to spirulina, a high-protein algae that contains omega-3
and omega-6 fatty acids, B-12 (important for vegetarians),
enzymes, and minerals. It also supports the immune system, fights
cancer, and helps with hypoglycemia, anemia, ulcers, diabetes, and
chronic fatigue syndrome. Spirulina also contains all nine essential
amino acids.[149]

Amino acids, huh? Yep. There are twenty amino acids. Our bodies produce eleven, and the other nine essential amino acids can be
obtained through food. Amino acids are the building blocks of protein. And yes, protein does build muscle. But even if you work out
and want to build muscle, you don't need to overdose on animal

protein (a ridiculous myth perpetuated by the health club industry). Bear in mind, some top athletes are vegetarians: Chris Campbell is an Olympic wrestling champion; Keith Holmes, a world-champion middleweight boxer; Bill Mannetti, a power-lifting champion; Bill Pearl, a four-time Mr. Universe; Andres Cahling, a champion body-builder and Olympic gold medalist in the ski jump; Art Still, a Hall of Famer and MVP defensive end for the NFL; Martina Navratilova, a tennis champion; and Dr. Ruth Heidrich, a six-time Ironwoman, age-group record holder, USA track and field Master's Champion, and vegan.[150]

Another common myth that has since been debunked is the "food combining" theory. Animal flesh proteins are "complete," meaning they contain all nine essential amino acids in amounts similar to those found in human flesh. Plants have all these amino acids, too, just in slightly different amounts. It was previously believed that in order to create complete proteins from vegetarian foods, you needed to combine them in specific ways. For example, it was said rice and beans had to be eaten together to maximize their protein potential. However, it is now known that eating a variety of foods from plant sources provides all the building blocks we need. Further, the microorganisms and recycled cells in our intestinal tracts make complete proteins for us.[151] All we have to do is eat healthy, balanced diets.

An integral part of any healthy, balanced diet is fat. Don't cringe. Fat doesn't always mean fattening. Essential fatty acids provide us with energy and offer protection from heart disease, stroke, and high blood pressure. They also combat allergies, premenstrual syndrome, arthritis, and skin problems.[152] Our brilliant bodies make all the essential fatty acids we need, except for two: linoleic and linolenic acids, also known as omega-3 and omega-6.[153] These *good fats* are found in olive oil, sesame oil, canola oil, flaxseed oil, hempseed oil, evening primrose oil, raw nuts and seeds, and avocados. So quit listening to all the stupid bitches who boycott nuts, oils, and avocados because they think they're fattening. Even though they're high in fat, they will not make you fat (unless you totally overdose on them). Unsaturated fats such as these are good for your body, and when eaten as part of a well-balanced vegan diet, they don't make you fat! It's the saturated fats, found in meat, dairy, and hydrogenated oils that make you fat. Think about the source of the oils or fats and use your head. Do you think an avocado, which is a fruit, is going to turn you into a hippo? Common sense, bitches.

Chapter 8

Pooping

Pinch a loaf. Lay cable. Drop the kids off at the pool. Let's face it; there is no greater pleasure than taking a big, steamy dump. But shitting isn't just for kicks. It is a vital tool for weight loss and optimal health. Basic math, girls. How much are you putting in your mouth, and how much is coming out your ass? Now that you've learned the right foods to eat and which ones to avoid, you should be a dynamo in the bathroom. But if your hiney is only expelling little rabbit turds, something's gotta give.

Earlier, we mentioned that drinking lots of water helps rid your body of waste. We can't emphasize the importance of this enough. Drink, drink, drink. But if you want to take tyrannosaurus-sized dumps, it's also imperative to eat foods rich in fiber, like whole grain cereals and breads, brown rice, corn, barley, rye, buckwheat, millet, oats, fruits, vegetables (especially root vegetables, like carrots), beans, and seeds. Avoid foods that have little or no fiber, like meat, eggs, cheese, milk, and processed, refined foods. These can clog up your ass. (It is a myth that bananas are binding. Eat 'em.)

Fiber isn't just for shits and giggles, either. It offers protection from appendicitis, Candida, heart disease, high blood pressure, high cholesterol, diabetes, gallstones, irritable bowel syndrome (IBS), and colitis.[154] Fibrous foods also help normalize our blood-sugar levels, satiate food cravings, and make us feel fuller so that we don't overeat.[155] Fiber even fights colon and colorectal cancer, prostate cancer, and breast cancer: If we don't make ca-ca quickly enough, our putrefying food stays in our bodies, increasing the likelihood of the production of carcinogenic substances. [156] So eat your fiber, and crap like a champ.

Another way to get your bowels brewing is to pay special attention to the order in which you are eating foods. For example, foods that digest quickly and easily should be eaten by themselves and early in the day. Fruit for breakfast. Salad and/or vegetables for lunch. These foods will pass through your body at lightning speeds. Dinner should be your "heaviest" meal. Follow these simple rules and you'll be depositing six-inchers in no time. If you're already a quality dumper, feel free to disregard this paragraph.

But, if you still need an extra kick in the ass, up your bean intake. Beware: you might have a mudslide in your pants if you're not careful. If you're not accustomed to beans, ease in slowly and be sure you are near a toilet.

If your deuce-dropping still needs work, do not take laxatives. Yes, they make you poop, but they don't solve the underlying problem of why you're not pooping in the first place. Most laxatives are gastro-intestinal irritants—even the natural ones.[157] Stop looking for a quick fix. Just continue to drink a lot of water, exercise, and eat right, shitheads.

Chapter 9

Have No Faith: Governmental Agencies Don't Give a Shit About Your Health

The USDA: It's Not What You Think

President Abraham Lincoln founded the U.S. Department of Agriculture in 1862—when the majority of people were farmers and needed to exchange information about seeds and crops. In other words, the USDA was created to help farmers.

According to its web site, now, among other things, the USDA is responsible for "the safety of meat, poultry, and egg products."[158]

Hmm. That's weird. 'Cause many high-ranking staff members at the USDA were employed by, or are otherwise affiliated with, the meat and dairy industries.[159] And if the group responsible for "the safety of meat, poultry, and egg products" is run by people from the same industries they're supposed to be protecting us from . . . well, that would be a conflict of interest. *And it is.* An enormous, ridiculous, outrageous, catastrophic conflict of interest.

One former USDA Secretary was forced to resign amid charges of accepting illegal corporate gifts from seven different companies. He was indicted on thirty-nine felony counts, including tampering with a witness; accepting illegal gratuities; making false statements; and violating the Meat Inspection Act of 1907. (Tyson Foods, one of the companies that admitted to giving the Secretary corporate favors, was required to pay $4 million in fines and endure four years' probation. A mere slap on the wrist, when the USDA could've barred Tyson from selling food to military bases and schools. That would've really stung, considering Tyson sold more than $10 million worth of food to the Defense Department alone in 1996.[160] But friends don't treat each other that way.)

President George W. Bush's Agriculture Secretary from January 2001 until January 2005, Ann Veneman, not only had ties with the company responsible for producing the controversial bovine growth hormone, (BGH), but she was also linked to a major meatpacking corporation.[161] The buck doesn't stop there. She employed a spokeswoman who was the former public relations director for the Cattlemen's Beef Association, a chief of staff who used to be its head lobbyist, a former president of the National Pork Producers Council, and former executives from the meatpacking industry, just to name a few.[162]

Safety Last

With that in mind, it's no wonder Veneman vetoed a program that would test all U.S. cattle for mad cow disease. In fact, out of the 35 million cattle slaughtered in 2003, the USDA only tested 20,000 for mad cow disease. (Japan tests *all* of their cattle killed for human consumption.)[163] Of course it wouldn't be in a rancher's best interest to test all of his cattle. If they were inflicted with mad cow disease, he couldn't sell their meat, and he'd lose money. Heaven forbid the USDA risk a rancher's profits.

So, in order to appear somewhat concerned about the prevention of mad cow disease, the USDA often refers to an FDA ban, which prohibits the feeding of ground-up cattle meat to live cattle. Big whoop. Banning cannibalism is a no-brainer. But why even bother banning cannibalism when they still allow the feeding of *cattle blood* to young calves? Stanley Prusiner, a Nobel Prize Winner for his work on mad cow disease, refers to this practice as "a really stupid idea."[164] Think about it: A cow dies from mad cow disease, but no one knows, because it wasn't one of the .0005714% percent tested. Cattle ranchers are now forbidden to grind up this dead cow and feed it to other cows. But, they can give its blood to calves as part of their feed. How fucking stupid, disgusting, and dangerous is that?

The USDA also likes referring to another "safety" program in place, called The National Animal Identification System (NAIS). The NAIS is a system for identifying an animal's origin so that if its meat is found to be contaminated, it can be traced back to a specific farm. (Forget testing as a preventative measure. Implement a system for after someone eats contaminated meat and we need a recall.) Participation in this program is voluntary.[165] Wow, the USDA sure has tough rules governing the safety of our country's meat.

The USDA's web site describing the NAIS actually has a section on "confidentiality." It reads, "The NAIS will contain only information necessary for animal health officials to be able to track suspect animals and identify any other animals that may have been exposed to a disease. . . . To help assure participants that the information will be used only for animal health purposes, the information must be confidential. USDA and its State partners will work to protect data confidentiality."[166] What the fuck? The USDA will protect the data confidentiality of farms that are supplying the public with contaminated meat? Why don't they just give all the ranchers blowjobs, too?

Many savvy consumers are catching on, and they know they cannot trust the USDA. According to the Organic Consumers Association, "Lester Friedlander, a former USDA veterinarian, says he was told by USDA officials as far back as 1991 that if his testing ever found evidence of Mad Cow disease, he was to tell no one. He and other scientists say they know of cases where cows tested positive for the disease in laboratories but were ruled negative by the USDA."[167] Trust no one!

Illegal hormones are regularly pumped into veal calves, which are suspected of increasing the growth of cancer cells in the humans who eat them. The USDA has not only been accused of overlooking these practices, but also of falsifying lab results, altering records, and pressuring staff to lie about events.[168] Even the selfish whores who eat veal don't deserve that.

Business First

None of us deserved to be deceived all these years by the preposterous USDA Dietary Guidelines and Food Pyramid, either. In 1998, the Physicians Committee for Responsible Medicine (PCRM) filed a federal lawsuit against the USDA and the Department of Health and Human Services. PCRM claimed that federal laws were violated when the USDA selected six out of eleven people with financial ties to various food industries to serve on the Dietary Guidelines Advisory Committee. The committee members' affiliations included the American Meat Institute,

National Livestock and Beef Board, the American Egg Board, the National Dairy Promotion and Research Program, the National Dairy Council, Dannon Company (yogurt), Mead Johnson Nutritionals (milk-based infant formulas), Nestlé (milk-based formulas, ice cream, condensed milk), and Slim-Fast (milk-based diet products).[169] How dare they?

(On a sidenote, PCRM also charged that the Dietary Guidelines —which recommended dairy products—were racially biased, because most nonwhites are lactose-intolerant.[170] According to Johnson & Johnson, lactose intolerance affects "over 50 percent of the Hispanic American population, 75 percent of Native Americans, 80 percent of African Americans, and 90 percent of Asian Americans."[171] Why does Johnson & Johnson care about the millions of minorities suffering from lactose intolerance? Because they can target these individuals for buying Lactaid, a product they hawk for aiding in dairy digestion. Even though you are lactose intolerant and your body thoroughly rejects dairy products, eat them anyway. Just buy and take our drug so you don't feel sick afterwards. Ugh, that just makes us sick with rage.)

Got $19 billion? The milk industry does, so they've got the USDA in their back pocket.[172] The California Milk Processor Board

(CMPB) was established in 1993 to increase milk sales in California. They were responsible for the campaigns that targeted children: "Got milk?" and "Milk. It does a body good." The CMPB is funded by all California milk processors, but administered by the California Department of Food and Agriculture. The National Fluid Milk Processor Promotion Board (Fluid Board) conceived of the "Milk Mustache" campaign, which targets young adults. The USDA's Agriculture Monitoring Service administers the Fluid Board.[173] Meaning, in essence, the California Department of Agriculture and the USDA are managing advertising campaigns for the milk industry. Under the guise of advancing health, they managed to dupe President Bill Clinton, while he was in office, into posing for their ads. They also had the audacity to feature the Secretary of Health and Human Services, Donna Shalala, sporting that stupid "milk mustache."[174] The Secretary of Health and Human Services using her status and title to promote a commercial product! Would she appear in ads for Pepsi or Nike? Say it out loud: conflict of interest. They've even got the U.S. surgeon general in on the act. In the first-ever report on "the state of the nation's bones," the U.S. surgeon general warned of an impending "osteoporosis crisis" expected by the year 2020. In order to ward off this potential disaster, the Surgeon General's report recommended three glasses of milk a day. Guess who issued the report? The Department of Health and Human Services.[175] Trust no one.

The horrors committed by the USDA could fill an entire book. But we shouldn't be surprised. Although they don't list it as part of their primary mission statement, the USDA does admit to being "committed to helping America's farmers and ranchers."[176] The same USDA responsible for "the safety" of meat, poultry, dairy, and eggs also promotes the sale of them. In fact, they even go so far as to purchase the products themselves, using *our* tax dollars. The USDA will spend $30 million a year on beef buyouts alone. Another $30 million of *our* hard-earned money goes toward pork purchases.[177] Wow. It must be nice for these industries to have the USDA bailing them out whenever they have a surplus of items. What, exactly, do they do with all this food that *we* pay for?

All in a Day's Work

Ever hear of the National School Lunch Program (NSLP)? It's a nation-wide $4 billion scheme that allows the USDA to buy up all this meat, milk, and cheese with our tax dollars, and then dump this crap into the bodies of more than 26 million school children.[178] Ever wonder why school lunches are *required* to include milk? The NSLP directly benefits the meat, dairy, and poultry industries at the expense of our nation's children.

In 1999, a ground beef plant in Texas failed a series of USDA tests for salmonella. The tests showed that as much as 47 percent of the company's ground beef contained salmonella—a proportion 5 times higher than what USDA regulations allow. Despite this, and the fact that high levels of salmonella in ground beef indicate high levels of fecal contamination, the USDA continued to purchase thousands of tons of the meat for distribution in schools. In fact, this company was one of the nation's largest suppliers for the school meals, providing as much as 45 percent of the program's ground meat.[179]

Contamination aside, according to Michele Simon of the Center for Informed Food Choices, "One evaluation of the commodity foods program estimates that 70 percent of the items offered exceed the U.S. dietary guidelines for fat."[180] For decades, consumer advocacy groups have been horrified by this unhealthy, profit-driven arrangement. With the backing of countless parents, physicians, and nutritionists, they have battled to get soy milk and other healthier choices approved by the USDA for use in school lunches. But the USDA (a.k.a.: the beef, pork, poultry, and dairy industries) wants no part in this, of course.

The USDA has fifteen food-assistance programs, including ones for the elderly, homeless, military, and poor. It is estimated that one in five Americans will take part in this $41.6 billion program.[181] Sounds like the USDA is helping to feed a lot of people, right? Right. They are feeding them fattening, unhealthy, artery-clogging, heart-stopping, acid-producing, contaminated meat, poultry, and dairy—with our money. How generous.

Organic or Not?

It's not enough that they dictate all things meat and dairy, the USDA even sticks its big nose into our organic products, too. In April 2004, the USDA made sweeping changes to their National Organic Program (NOP) standards. The new rules infuriated organic farmers and consumers because: Livestock were allowed to eat non-organic fishmeal, even if it contained toxins or synthetic preservatives; cows and calves given growth hormones, antibiotics, or other drugs could still provide the public with "organic" milk, as long as a year had passed since the drugs were administered; pesticides could be used even if they contained unknown inert ingredients as long as a "reasonable effort" had been made to identify them; and seafood, pet food, clothing, fertilizers, and body care products could be labeled organic without being monitored by the USDA.[183] Not only were people livid with the actual changes, but also with the decision-making process. By law, these types of regulatory changes are required to undergo a period of public comment before being enacted. There was no comment period, just an announcement of changes after the fact.[184]

According to Ronnie Cummins, national director of Organic Consumers Association (OCA), "Rather than comply with regulations which uphold the integrity of organic food, corporate-run factory farms, who want a piece of the $11 billion a year organic industry, are manipulating the USDA and Congress to change the rules to suit their toxic-industrial style of farming. Allowing non-organic, and potentially genetically engineered feed to be included under the definition of "organic" is a major setback for the integrity of what is the fastest-growing sector of the food industry in this country."[185] Thanks to the phone calls, letters, e-mails, and faxes of many pissed off consumers, the USDA reversed all these changes in May 2004.[186]

Even so, many people are still mistrustful of the USDA. Nonprofit group, The Center for Food Safety (CFS), claims that the USDA may be allowing "sham" certifiers under the umbrella of the National Organic Program (NOP). Their suspicions were aroused by the high volume of certifications issued within a short time. These worries were heightened when the USDA refused to provide CFS with requested documents, even though they were required to do so under the Freedom of Information Act.[187]

Other environmental groups along with the OCA have joined a lawsuit against the USDA. Among their complaints was the fact that the USDA's NOP created an additional category of certified products, which directly opposes legislation put in place by Congress. They state, "When Congress has spoken clearly on a subject, USDA has no discretion to rewrite the statute making exceptions that dilute the standards of the Act."[188] Can you believe the nerve of these USDA fuckers? Going against laws created by our elected officials and making up their own rules? It's fucking mutiny, is what it is. Trust no one.

When buying organic foods, look for certification from anyone other than the USDA. Oregon Tilth, California Certified Organic Farmers, Marin Organic Certifying Agency, and Demeter Certified Biodynamic are all reputable. Sometimes a product will be certified organic by the USDA and another party. So don't rule it out just because the USDA certifies it.

Surely you've seen the "organic" Horizon brand of dairy products in your grocery store? It is the nation's largest supplier of organic dairy products. Well, it just so happens that Horizon has been accused of violating organic standards. The Cornucopia Institute, a watchdog group in support of organic agriculture, filed two complaints with the USDA. They allege that two major farms that supply Horizon with milk are confining cows in an industrial setting and denying them access to pasture, yet are still calling their products organic.[189]

Why is all this allowed to happen? Don't our elected officials know what's going on? Why don't they try to stop this? Some do. But many politicians are in bed with the evil industries. McDonald's alone has made close to $2 million in campaign contributions; the National Cattlemen's Beef Association nearly $1.5 million; and the National Restaurant Association more than $3.1 million.[190] Hate to sound like a broken record player, but trust no one.

Is Everyone in the FDA on Drugs?

This greed-induced immorality isn't applicable just to Congress or the USDA. The Food and Drug Administration (FDA) is a pathetic facade, too. In 1990, the Monsanto Company sought FDA approval for Posilac, a commercialized form of bovine growth hormone (BGH, used to increase cows' milk production). Even though the test study linked the hormone to prostate and thyroid cancer, the FDA still approved Posilac. Of course, these damning test results weren't made available to the public until 1998, when a group of scientists conducted an independent analysis of the study. They found that the FDA never even reviewed Monsanto's findings! More recently, BGH has been linked to increased levels of Insulin Growth Factor-1, a cancer promoter. But the FDA has no interest in these findings, either. Or the fact that both the World Trade Organization and The United Nations Food Standards Body refuse to endorse the hormone's safety. And they certainly don't mind that BGH milk is banned in all of the European Union, Canada, Japan, and every other industrialized country in the world.[191] Fucking Dumb Asses.

Why would the FDA knowingly allow a cancer-causing hormone into our milk supply? One theory highlights the fact that the FDA Deputy Commissioner at the time of the Posilac approval was a former Monsanto lawyer. And, during his tenure at the FDA, this same deputy commissioner wrote the policy exempting BGH from special labeling. Yet, fingers also point to a former top scientist with Monsanto, who was hired by the FDA to review her *own* research, conducted while she was working for Monsanto. This little beauty also allowed a hundred-fold increase of antibiotic residues in milk.[192]

Fear not. The FDA's bad behavior isn't singular to the dairy industry. It also has a sketchy history with monosodium glutamate (MSG). One former FDA Commissioner testified before the Senate Select Committee on Nutrition that MSG was safe, citing four sources. It was later discovered that two of the studies were nonexistent, and the other two were incomplete![193]

Secrets and lies. It's just too much to bear. So let's also play the "I'm not telling" game. Ever see the words "natural flavors" on food packaging ingredient lists? Yeah, that's because the FDA allows companies to be vague and doesn't require them to tell us exactly what we're eating. The FDA has a list of approximately 300 foods that meet a "standard of identity," meaning, companies aren't required to spell out their ingredients. For example, ice cream manufacturers can use any of twenty-five specified additives without listing them in their ingredients.[194] Who wants to put something into his or her body without even knowing what it is? By now, Chapter 9, *you* better fucking not!

You Are Your Only Chance

If you want to get skinny, you can only rely on yourself. If you adapt only one practice from this book, let it be this: *Read the ingredients.* Forget counting carbs, adding calories, and multiplying fat grams. Just read the ingredients. It doesn't matter how many calories or carbs or fat grams something has. *It just doesn't matter.* You don't need the government's asinine recommended daily allowances (RDA) to tell you how to eat. Just read the ingredients. If they are healthy, wholesome, and pure—dive in. If there is refined sugar, white or bleached flour, hydrogenated oils, any animal products, artificial anything, or some scary-looking word that you don't know—don't eat it. We can't make it any simpler. Just read the ingredients and completely ignore all the other gibber jabber bullshit the government calls for on the packaging. Fuck them. Trust no one. Get skinny.

And no matter what, do not fall prey to clever advertising used on the packaging. The companies that call their products "wholesome" or "nutritious" can be the same ones that add hydrogenated oils, artificial flavors, or synthetic preservatives. Just read the ingredients of everything you buy. It's not a big deal, assuming you are literate.

There is so much bureaucracy and red tape surrounding health-related government agencies that you are much better off fending for yourself. After all, why would anyone take nutritional advice from organizations that let color dyes, hydrogenated oils, chemical preservatives, and artificial flavors into the food we eat?

The EPA Makes Us Sick

StarLink corn, a genetically modified organism, contains an insecticidal protein, deemed unsafe for human consumption. But the Environmental Protection Agency allows the use of StarLink for livestock feed.[195] Let humans eat the animals who ate the corn? That's safe? Duh.

Clearly, nothing is sacred to the group that allows *rocket fuel* in our milk supply. Yeah, you heard right. Rocket fuel. In milk. Thanks to the Pentagon, ammonium perchlorate, the main explosive component in rocket fuel, has been lurking around our environment for decades. It finds its way into water used for growing feed crops for cattle. Cows eat these contaminated crops, with the result being contaminated milk. Whether you are drinking milk or eating dairy products made with this milk, you are ingesting perchlorate. And the EPA actually makes allowances for a "provisional daily safe dose."[196] We're sorry, but where we're from—Earth—there is no acceptable amount to ingest where explosive components are concerned. Even if you believe any amount to be safe, tests revealed milk perchlorate levels well above the EPA's index. Studies conducted by the Environmental Working Group (EWG), a nonprofit, non-partisan organization, found *every single* milk sample tested in Texas to be contaminated. California's own Food and Agriculture Department found that milk off the grocers' shelves had *five times* the EPA's "safe dose" of perchlorate. But, of course, the California Food and Agriculture Department did not release these results. Instead, they were brought to light by the EWG. Although both the dairy industry and government agencies acknowledge that there could be some health risks associated with perchlorate, they maintain that we should keep drinking milk for its "calcium, protein and minerals."[197] We'll let you use your own heads on this one.

Regardless of your political affiliation, please know this: The Bush Administration continuously asks for exemptions on behalf of the military and chemical companies, allowing them to continue this contamination and to shirk responsibility for cleanup. In fact, the Bush administration's EPA has been widely criticized on many counts of environmental pollution that affect our food and water supply. Like the USDA's pathetic voluntary program, the EPA has its own version of letting agribusiness trample all over public health and safety. Collaborating closely with the U.S. Poultry and Egg Association and

The National Pork Producers Council (NPPC), the EPA developed a *voluntary* air-monitoring program. Disregard the notion that the EPA blames factory farming for 73 percent of all ammonia (fumes from all the shit and piss of farm animals) released into the air nationwide. Never mind the fact that the EPA names factory farming to be the single largest contributor of polluted American waterways. Factory farmers do not have to submit to EPA monitoring programs.[198] If it pleases them, they can volunteer. How civilized.

Outraged by the EPA's lack of enforcement, opponents point out that the factory farming industry made $3.46 million in campaign contributions, benefiting mostly Republican federal candidates. The NPPC even went so far as to present President Bush with its "Friend of the Pork Producer" award in 2004, thanking him for his help in "shaping environmental policies impacting agriculture." [199] Yeah, um, thanks for that.

Trust No One

Whether you love him or hate him, President Clinton's administration tried to "implement a tough, science-based food inspection system," according to Eric Schlosser, bestselling author of *Fast Food Nation*. Sad to say, however, these attempts were squashed when the Republican party gained control of Congress in 1994. Schlosser revealed, "The meatpacking industry's allies in Congress worked hard to thwart modernization of the nation's meat inspection system. A great deal of effort was spent denying the federal government any authority to recall contaminated meat or impose civil fines on firms that knowingly ship contaminated products. . . . . The Clinton administration backed legislation to provide the USDA with the authority to demand meat recalls and impose civil fines on meatpackers. [But] Republicans in Congress failed to enact not only that bill, but also similar legislation [for four consecutive years.] . . . Under current law, the USDA cannot demand a recall [of contaminated meat.]" Can you fucking believe this? If a company decides voluntarily to recall contaminated meat, "it is under no legal obligation to inform the public—or even health officials—that a recall is taking place." [200]

Now, we don't mean to say that everyone working for the government is evil. Surely there are some decent, caring, moral, intelligent, well-intentioned people working for the FDA, EPA,

USDA, and Bush administration. One former staff attorney-turned-environmentalist said the EPA "hasn't initiated one investigation in four years. They're not doing anything."[201] See, she's a "good guy!" She finked on the EPA. Unfortunately, many of the "good guys" seem to be lost in the shuffle of politics and greed within these groups.

So do yourself a favor and trust no one. Read ingredients. Ignore everything else. And, if you're totally incensed by what you've just learned, do something. Contact your representatives, senators, the President and Vice President and demand reform of these crooked, self-serving agencies. Go to www.congress.org to send a quick e-mail to these politicians. While you're at it, write a letter to the editor of your favorite magazine or newspaper, and ask others to join the crusade. Visit www.congress.org and click on "media guide" to access their contact information.

Chapter 10

Don't Be a Pussy

What if someone told you that you could totally change your life and have the body you want for the rest of your life? What if all you had to do was follow a simple formula and maybe struggle for a month or two? What if you could reprogram your brain to actually enjoy healthy foods? Well, guess what? You *can* change your life. You *can* have the body you want for the rest of your life. You *can* enjoy healthy foods. All you have to do is follow a simple formula, and be willing to delay gratification for a few months. A few months. That's it. Then you can enjoy a new body for the *rest of your life.* Don't be a pussy. You have all the nutritional information you need to become a Skinny Bitch. The rest is up to you. While this is a lifestyle, and not a diet, it is going to feel like a diet for the first thirty days or so. During this time, you will be retraining your brain, healing your taste buds, and cleansing and detoxifying your body. It might suck a little. Chances are, there will be times you feel deprived, angry, overwhelmed, and frustrated. But these few, fleeting moments will all be worthwhile once you are skinny. Truth be told, if you follow our guidelines, it won't be so bad.

Before you even start making changes, take notice of how you feel and the role that your diet plays. Do you wake up tired? Is coffee the only thing that gets you going in the morning? Are you cranky in the afternoon? Do you need snacks to bolster your mood? Do you have little or no energy? Do you rely on soda or sugar for a little boost? Do you have trouble falling asleep? Is a glass of wine the only thing that gets you drowsy? When you eat something unhealthy, how do you feel while you're eating it? Right after? An hour later? How does it affect your sleep that night? How do you feel the next day? Pay attention to the negative effects your current diet and lifestyle have on your body, moods, and energy level. Feel free to start a little journal, writing what you eat and drink throughout the day and how you feel as a result. This way, when you start making positive changes to your diet, you'll appreciate *all* of the results—not just the weight loss.

Recognize that anything worth having is worth fighting for. Good health, vitality, more energy, more confidence, better sex, great abs, a tight ass—you either want 'em or you don't. You can continue plodding along in your life feeling like you're not living up to your glorious potential or you can dedicate yourself to creating the life you want. Fuck excuses about not having the time or the money. You spend forty hours a week working, or more if you're a full-time mom. Certainly your health and your body and *you* are more important than anything else in your life. You are worthless to your colleagues, friends, and family if you do not value yourself enough to take excellent care of *you*. Yes, you have to put *yourself* before your friends, parents, boyfriend, husband, and even your children. It won't make you a bad daughter or wife or mother; it will make you a less resentful, more confident, interesting, beautiful, patient, tolerant, and fun person to be around. Your bright, shining light will give everyone around you the permission and inspiration to shine more brightly. Love yourself enough to do whatever it takes to be the best *you* you can be.

An important part of any recovery program for addiction—and unhealthy eating is an addiction—is taking one day at a time. Don't torture yourself with thoughts of, "I can never eat steak again," or "How will I live without coffee?" Just take it one meal at a time. Don't think ahead with dread and anguish. One meal at a time. And when all feels hopeless, remember that you are in charge of what goes into your body, you don't answer to anyone, and you are *allowed* to eat anything you want. Often just knowing we *can* eat whatever we want is enough to keep us from eating whatever we want. We're so rebellious.

If you feel really invigorated and motivated, and you're ready to completely immerse yourself in the Skinny Bitch lifestyle now, then rock on. Go for it. Otherwise, feel free to set mini-goals for yourself and tackle them one at a time. This means, spend the first week of your new life removing one dirty vice item. Whether it's cigarettes or coffee or alcohol or sugar or junk food or meat or dairy—just purge something negative from your life immediately. Choose something that you like and enjoy, but that you know you can let go of successfully. (But start right now. Don't let these intense feelings fade—use them.) Dedicate the week to getting this vice item out of your diet, your body, your kitchen, and your mind. Think of all you've learned about this item, and how disgusting it is. Envision the damaging effect it has on your organs, your mood, your health, and your appearance. Imagine exactly what it is that you'd be eating. Know how shitty you'd feel, physically and mentally, if you ate it. Understand that you have free will and that if you *wanted* to eat it, you could. But know with every fiber and cell of your being that *today* you wish to put only pure, beautiful, healthful foods in your body. Most important, acknowledge that no vice item will ever make you feel happy or whole or satisfied. In fact, all vice items make you *unhappy* because they contribute to weight issues, health problems, mood swings, and low self-esteem.

When you've got one week under your belt, feel great about what you've accomplished. Then, immediately, while continuing to steer clear of the item you banished in week one, start week two by ridding something else from your diet. Every week, until you've completely cleansed your life of poison and toxins, eliminate one more thing. Apply the same mindset, dedication, technique, and excitement you used in week one. Resign yourself to purifying your thoughts, body, and kitchen of this crappy vice item; realize you've just made your life better by not letting this vice item infect you anymore; gross yourself out thinking about what exactly it is and the effects it has on your body; think of how bad it makes you feel when you partake in it; and finally, remember that if you did *choose* to eat/smoke/drink it, it wouldn't make you happy or fulfilled.

Never feel like or say you are "giving up" your favorite foods. Those words have a negative connotation, like you are sacrificing something. You're not *giving up* anything. You are simply empowered now and able to make educated, controlled choices about what you will and won't put into your body, your temple. Be grateful that you now know the truth about the foods you used to poison yourself with. Let all you think and speak of regarding this life change be positive. People who have positive attitudes are much more successful than those who don't. Be excited about feeling clean, pure, healthy, energized, happy, and skinny. Enjoy every second of this metamorphosis, knowing the journey is as important as the end result.

Confucius never said, "A hungry woman is like a tornado of red ants and wildebeasts," but he should have. Because it's true. A hungry woman is a crazy woman, who will destroy everything in her path to be rid of the hunger. So you must always be prepared with healthy food on hand. Otherwise, seriously, you will fall off the wagon almost immediately. Your kitchen should be stocked at all times with the appropriate foods. Pack your lunch and a snack for school or work. Keep an emergency stash in your car, at your desk, and in your purse. Never, ever get caught with your pants down. Unfortunately, depending on where you live, restaurants may not be a safe place for the first month. The menu might not have any vegan or even vegetarian options, and it is easy to be hypnotized by the seductive smells of cooking. This doesn't mean you can't eat out ever again as long as you live. Just for thirty days. (Unless there are good veggie-friendly restaurants in your neighborhood.) You can't expect to change your life without a few minor adjustments. Your only priority for thirty days is to adhere to the regimen you're creating. Without straying. After you achieve thirty days of pure eating, you'll feel confident you have what it takes to get the job done. "I just survived thirty days. I'm so proud of myself. This is the healthiest I've ever been in my whole life. If I *want* to, I can eat an old vice item. But why would I? I just made it thirty consecutive days. I'm going to keep going." If you test yourself before thirty days, you are setting yourself up for failure. Be patient and strong.

When you reach the thirty-day milestone, don't run out and gorge yourself on crap. In fact, just keep doing what you've been doing. See and feel all the positive changes in your body, energy level, and self-esteem. Alcohol, cigarettes, coffee, and food are all addictive, physically and psychologically. Chances are, even after the thirty days, if you indulge in a vice item, you might go off the deep end. It is well known in Alcoholics Anonymous that you're only "one drink away from your next drunk." This means we think we can control our addictions. "I'll just have one drink. I'll just have pizza this one time. I'll just eat half a piece of cake." The truth of the matter is that we are powerless over our addictions. We don't want to make you feel like you can never eat your favorite foods ever again. We just want to impress upon you that it is very easy to obliterate all your progress with one bite, sip, or puff.

Anyway, after one month of pure living, if you did eat the food you've been fantasizing about, you probably wouldn't even enjoy it. Really. You'd see that your brain has been tricking you and your taste buds all along. Now that your taste buds have healed and become more sensitized and your brain knows the truth, those old chemical, sugary, artificial, dead, rotting foods will taste "off" or "less than" somehow.

If you do decide to partake in a vice item after thirty days, it cannot be out of weakness or for lack of preparation. You should never be somewhere and just say, "Fuck it." It should be a calculated, scheduled, premeditated choice. The portion should be decided on beforehand, should be smaller than you would normally have had, and served on a plate. (The package should be put away before you start eating.) Sit down at a table. Eat very slowly. Try not to finish the whole thing. Do not have another serving. Take note of how you feel while you're eating it, immediately after, an hour later, in bed that night, and the next day. Chances are, because your body is now pure, the vice item will make you feel a little nauseous, or headache-y, at the very least. And it most certainly won't taste as good as you imagine it will. Do not discount these negative feelings. They are your new, healthy, clean, pure organs speaking to you.

Enough of all this melodrama. It's not like you're gonna be hungry and cranky for all of eternity. We know that dieters always "crash" when their favorite foods become forbidden. So we devised the Skinny Bitch plan to allow for cookies, cakes, chocolate, burgers, ice cream, etc. They just aren't the same ones you're used to. You're not giving up anything; you're just trading in all your old, gross food. Big deal. The new stuff is just as good. So don't kid yourself with the old "I had a craving" routine. Nobody's buying it.

The only thing more annoying than the "Where do you get your protein?" question is the "My body is craving meat, I must need iron" comment. Most cravings are not reliable indicators of what your body needs. Smokers crave cigarettes, alcoholics crave alcohol, drug addicts crave drugs, and junk food eaters crave junk. If you eat shit for a few days, and you begin to crave a salad or a piece of fruit, that's a craving you can trust. Otherwise, it's just your addiction talking. Bitch-slap it, and get a hold of yourself. But feel free to try and understand your addiction first.

In order for us to survive, our brains came equipped with dopamine, a pleasure-producing chemical. Dopamine is released during sex (or even just while flirting), so that we procreate and the human race won't die out. And food stimulates dopamine release so that we'll remember to eat and nourish our bodies. Basically, anything the brain perceives to be enjoyable will cause dopamine to lock onto brain cells and build a permanent memory trace of where pleasure comes from. Even though this evolved out of the need for survival, sometimes this can be a bad thing. Heroin, cocaine, alcohol, and nicotine all trigger the brain's pleasure circuitry. And not surprisingly, chocolate, sugar, and cheese also affect this same part of the brain. So you see, we can be *physiologically* addicted to food. Any food can trigger the brain's pleasure center. Some of us are fortunate enough to experience dopamine ecstasy while eating broccoli, and we actually crave this healthy food. But the types of food and the degree of pleasure they bring will differ from one person to the next. The trick is resetting our memory traces to feel pleasure from healthy food, and no pleasure from junk food.[202]

Easier said than done. Especially for people who are addicted to cigarettes, alcohol, or drugs, or are overweight. Studies have shown that these people have fewer receptors for dopamine than other people. For them, the pleasure-giving chemical has fewer places to attach to brain cells, making it difficult for them to experience pleasurable feelings. So, because they aren't getting that "pleasure rush," they tend to smoke, drink, use drugs, gamble, or overeat. Now don't automatically diagnose yourself as one these people and assume you'll never get healthy. We are not at the mercy of our bodies. We are the commanders of our bodies.[203]

Unless we eat cheese. Cheese will rule our lives and fatten our asses if we don't kick the addiction. Cow's milk actually has traces of morphine in it! And for once, we can't blame factory farming. Morphine, along with codeine and other opiates, are naturally produced in cows' livers and end up in their milk. But that's not all. All milk, whether from a cow or a human, contains *casein,* a protein that breaks apart during digestion and releases a whole slew of opiates. All these "feel good" chemicals exist so that newborns will nurse and thrive, and to ensure a bond between mothers and their young.[204]

Are you starting to get the picture? When a woman breastfeeds, her milk has an almost drug-like effect on the baby. The baby is totally hooked. He'll cry, not because he's hungry, but because he needs "a fix" of that pleasurable feeling produced by the opiates. Nature has guaranteed that our babies will nurse and grow. And when they reach a certain age, we wean them, and stop giving them these "drugs." And they're fine. But then we start them on cows' milk and an addiction is born.

All dairy products contain casein, but cheese has the highest concentration. In fact, cheese contains far more casein than is naturally found in cows' milk. It also has phenylethylamine (PEA), an amphetamine-like chemical. So when we kid around and say, "I am addicted to cheese," it's not a joke—it's true. We are chemically addicted to cheese.[205]

Casein even finds its way into soy cheese. Whether manufacturers use it to up the protein content, to aide in melting, or because they know of its addictive quality, casein still has the same effect. So if you see casein on the list of ingredients, run! (Follow Your Heart's Vegan Gourmet cheeses are casein-free and totally vegan, so enjoy.)

The following hormones and natural chemicals have all been identified in cows' milk: prolactin, somatostatin, melatonin, oxytocin, growth hormone, leuteinizing hormone-releasing hormone, thyrotropin-releasing hormone, thyroid-stimulating hormone, vasoactive intestinal peptide, calcitonin, parathyroid hormone, corticosteroids, estrogens, progesterone, insulin, epidermal growth

factor, insulin-like growth factor, erythropoietin, bombesin, neu-
rotensin, motilin, and cholecystokinin.[206] If you think your will is
strong enough to conquer all those mother-fuckers, you're on
drugs! Dairy is fattening,[207] and if you eat it, you'll never get skinny.
You cannot control your addiction. You can't "just have one slice of
pizza," or "only have cheese at parties." You're only one piece-of-
cheese away from a total relapse. Eat the substitutes; they'll get you
through.

Thankfully, our bodies produce a few different chemical substances that help tame our appetites. One such hormone, leptin, is
made by our fat cells. When fat cells in our bodies get adequate
nourishment, they release leptin into the blood for two purposes.
The first task at hand is alerting the brain to diminish the appetite.
Next, our metabolism gets boosted, encouraging the body's cells to
burn calories more quickly. Pretty cool, huh? Until we start "diet-
ing." Typical low-calorie diets confuse the body into thinking it's
starving. So our fat cells slow down their leptin production, to help
increase our appetites. Release the hounds! Now, we feel like we're
starving! So we trash our diets and binge like rabid beasts. But diets
high in fat don't fare any better. Fatty diets (think animal products)

also lower leptin levels. You know where this is headed: Low-fat, plant-based diets actually boost leptin levels, helping each molecule of leptin to work more effectively. So help yourself succeed. Eating healthy foods like fruits, vegetables, whole grains, and beans will help curb your appetite and stimulate your metabolism.[208]

But when we have PMS, all bets are off. There's no telling when we'll cry, whom we'll kill, or what we'll eat. One culprit of mood swings and cravings is estrogen. Every month, our bodies produce extra estrogen in case of pregnancy. When we don't become preggers, estrogen levels plunge, triggering bloating, irritability, and cravings. The trick to avoiding these heinous feelings is maintaining balanced estrogen levels throughout the month. Like everything else, this can be done through diet. Fatty foods increase estrogen levels, while fibrous foods help reduce estrogen production. The *Journal of Obstetrics and Gynecology* conducted a study exploring the effects of diet on menstrual symptoms. Women who eliminated animal fats from their diets experienced dramatic decreases of bloating and cravings. On average, menstrual cramps were reduced from four days to about two and a half days.[209] Less cramps, cravings, and bloating! Those reasons alone are enough to swear off animal products.

Even if you do have some serious PMS cravings, the good thing about the Skinny Bitch regimen is that there are plenty of naughty-tasting foods that you don't need to feel bad about. So eat all day long. As long as everything you put in your mouth meets Skinny Bitch approval, it's fine. Just be sure that when you're full, you *stop eating*. We know this is a foreign concept, but we're hoping it'll catch on. Imagine the actual size of your stomach (about the size of a one-quart container) or imagine what size you want it to be. There is no need to cram it full and stretch the shit out of it three times a day, every day, for your entire life. Look at the portion you put on your plate. Do you think it will fit in your stomach nicely, or that you'll need to force it in? Pare down.

Just because you're "starving," you don't need to eat faster. When you're done eating, if you have the hiccups, indigestion, a stomachache, or you're burping and farting, that means you're eating too fast and gulping down air. Slow down. Breathe evenly. Conversely, make sure you aren't holding your breath while you speed-eat. It takes time for your brain to get the message that your stomach is full. The slower you eat, the less likely you are to overeat. Also, be sure to chew your food purposefully and slowly. Rest in between bites. Do not watch TV, read a magazine, talk on the phone, or do *anything else* while you are eating. The goal is to know when you're full (without having *stuffed* yourself) and be able to put the fork down. You aren't six anymore. You won't get the praise of elders for cleaning your plate. It's okay to leave food on your plate.

But if you do still get off on scoring brownie points, you can earn extra credit by fasting. Yeah, fasting—willfully abstaining from food. For more than five thousand years, fasting has been used as a healthy method of weight loss. It is also a powerful tool for cleaning, flushing, detoxifying, and maintaining the body, and healing illnesses, both minor and major.[210] When we eat, all of our body's energy goes toward digesting, using, and storing the food, and eliminating the waste. When we don't eat, all of our body's energy goes toward cleaning house. And with all the years of abuse, our house could sure use a cleaning. We absorb toxic chemicals from food, drinks, and the environment. Our body eliminates some of these through waste, but the rest remain as chemical by-products and free radicals (highly reactive chemicals that damage cells and contribute to premature aging, heart disease, and cancer). Fasting gets rid of these toxins. It also increases our blood's white cell count, which boosts immunity and protects us from disease. And because fasting is beneficial for the circulatory system, you can expect better skin, hair, and nails.[211]

Fasts can last anywhere from twenty-four hours to ten days or more. It's all up to you and how light, clean, and healthy you want to get. The longer the better, but even just one day one time a month is beneficial. There are too many types of fasts to cover them all, so we'll explain just a few. But it is imperative to really read up on fasting before diving in.

A particular favorite is a raw or "live" food fast, when, obviously, you eat only raw foods for however many days you choose. This is a great beginner's fast, because you reap the benefits of fasting, while still being able to actually eat. It's also a good fast to do if you want to work your way up to a more stringent fast, like a juice fast, where the only thing you put in your body is fresh-pressed or fresh-squeezed juice (not pasteurized or packaged). Whether its fruit juice, veggie juice, or both, the enzymes are wonderful aides in the cleansing process. A liquid fast is similar to the juice fast, but includes soups,

too (no beans or rice or chunks—just liquid). The alkalizing properties of the juices and soups help to neutralize the toxins being
released from the body.[212] For this and other reasons, the hardest fast
is a water fast, where you have nothing but water. Don't be a competitive ass and launch yourself into this fast from the diet you exist on
now. You've gotta learn to crawl before you can walk.

Most people like to ease into a fast. They might eat smaller portions for a week prior. Or if they usually eat vegan junk food, they
might abstain in preparation. We highly recommend eating as pure-
ly as possible leading up to a fast. (Meat-eaters should go
vegetarian and then vegan before fasting.) It makes the transition
more gradual and less jarring. Regardless of which fast you choose,
be sure to drink a lot of water throughout. Your body will be detox-
ing like crazy, and you don't want to become dehydrated.

All fasts are challenging, both physically and mentally. Do not
expect it to be easy, especially at the beginning when you find yourself salivating over foods you don't normally even care about. But
eventually, you get to a place where you are truly not hungry, and
you feel light, clean, pure, and divine. When you do reintroduce
food back into your diet, which should be done slowly with great

care, you are almost repulsed by things you previously ate. It is quite beautiful to have such a new, fresh perspective. It is a real gift to see truths that weren't apparent before. Periodic repeated fasts are especially useful for this reason. They help our bodies and minds reestablish a new relationship with food. In fact, because of this, fasting can even be used to overcome addictions. When we eliminate the toxins that cause "cell memory cravings," we can eradicate the need for the food or drug that provided those toxins.[213]

Not surprisingly, some people experience headaches, weakness, nausea, cramping, stomach pains, sweating, a swollen tongue, bad breath, general aches and pains, increased temperature, or depression while fasting.[214] Abstaining from food does not *cause* these ailments. They are simply normal side effects of fasting. After two to three days of fasting, the body goes into autolysis, and actually starts digesting its own cells. With its wisdom, the body selectively decomposes the tissues and cells that are diseased, damaged, old, dead or in excess (fat).[215] The body is literally digesting and expelling poisons, toxins, and bad cells that were already there—and it feels crappy. But this is actually a good thing, because the body is finally able to tackle some problems that were lurking within.

During a fast, digestive enzymes are relieved from their usual role, and instead act to cleanse and rejuvenate the body. This rejuvenation process includes the production of new cells. And when more cells are being produced than are dying, the aging process is actually being reversed. This phenomenon occurs during juice and water fasts. Eventually, you'll notice sharper senses of smell, sight, sound, and taste. You'll feel lighter physically, mentally, and emotionally.[216]

All magic aside, fasting is *not* for you if you're pregnant, lactating, underweight, or suffering from severe wasting diseases, such as neurological degenerative diseases and certain cancers. Diabetics and people suffering from hypoglycemia can fast, but only with medical supervision.[217] For that matter, anyone with any medical condition should consult a doctor before fasting.

Vitamins

Vitamins are an integral part of a healthy lifestyle. Here are some significant vitamins and minerals, a description of why they're important, and which foods provide them:

Calcium strengthens bones, provides for healthy teeth, reduces risk

of colon cancer, decreases chances of bone loss, aids the
nervous system, and alleviates insomnia. Eat almonds, Brazil
nuts, seeds, nuts, soybeans, kale, collard greens, broccoli,
kelp, and molasses to get calcium.

Folic acid promotes healthy skin, protects against parasites and
food poisoning, helps ward off anemia, and fights against
birth defects. To get folic acid, eat leafy green veggies, carrots, artichokes, fruit, cantaloupe, avocados, apricots, beans,
lentils, soybeans, garbanzos, barley, and whole wheat.

Iron aids growth, promotes resistance to disease, prevents fatigue
and anemia, and enhances good skin tone. It can be found in
nuts, pumpkin seeds, beans, lentils, whole grains, oatmeal,
asparagus, molasses, broccoli, spinach, bok choy, peas, swiss
chard, green beans, and sea veggies.

Magnesium (known as the anti-stress mineral) fights depression,
boosts energy, helps burn fat, prevents heart attacks, maintains good cholesterol levels, aids indigestion, combats PMS
symptoms, helps prevent premature labor, and keeps teeth
strong and healthy. When combined with calcium, it works as
a natural tranquilizer. Eat nuts, seeds, sunflower seeds, green

vegetables, soybeans, kelp (seaweed), and molasses to get a good dose, especially if you're on The Pill.

Omega-3 fatty acids fight heart disease, lower bad cholesterol levels, lessen the likelihood of blood clots, reduce the risk of breast cancer, help with rheumatoid arthritis, and keep skin, hair, and nails healthy. Sources for these fatty acids are flaxseeds, walnuts, pumpkin seeds, hempseed oil, and other seeds and their unrefined oils.

Omega-6 fatty acids combat PMS, ward off acne, eczema, and psoriasis, and help with endometriosis and rheumatoid arthritis. Flaxseed oil, evening primrose oil, borage oil, and black currant seed oil are all good sources.

Potassium aids in reducing blood pressure, increases clear thinking by helping send oxygen to the brain, and helps the body dispose of waste. It's found in bananas, citrus fruits, cantaloupe, tomatoes, watercress, green leafy vegetables, sunflower seeds, avocados, lentils, potatoes, and whole grains.

The **B Vitamins** improve mental attitude, aid in digestion, help migraine headaches, contribute to healthy skin, act as natural

diuretics, strengthen immunity, increase energy, improve concentration and memory, and are good for the nervous system.
Eat whole wheat, wheat germ, bran, oatmeal, whole grains,
brown rice, beans, nuts, seeds, soybeans, lentils, dates, figs,
bananas, and vegetables.

Vitamin C accelerates healing, lowers blood pressure, prevents
colds, protects against cancer, and helps decrease blood cholesterol. It also forms collagen, which is important for growth
the and repair tissue cells, blood vessels, gums, bones, and
teeth. Vitamin C is especially important for women who
smoke or take birth control pills. It's easy to get vitamin C by
eating broccoli, brussel sprouts, cabbage, collard greens,
green peppers, spinach, watercress, potatoes, grapefruits,
oranges, and papayas.

Vitamin D, in conjunction with calcium and phosphorous, helps
build strong bones and teeth. Not only does vitamin D help
our bodies assimilate vitamin A, but it also prevents colds
when teamed up with vitamins A and C. All you need to do to
obtain vitamin D is get direct sun exposure on your skin.

Vitamin E keeps you looking younger, inhibits cancer cell growth, fights fatigue, prevents blood clots, lowers blood pressure, decreases the risk of Alzheimer's disease, and accelerates the healing of burns. It's found in wheat germ, whole grain cereals, whole wheat, nuts, sunflower seeds, leafy greens, and vegetable oils.

Zinc helps with infertility issues, is important for brain function, maintains the body's acid/alkaline balance, aids in collagen formation, and helps form insulin (needed for many vital enzymes). Foods with high concentrations of zinc are wheat germ, whole grains, pumpkin seeds, sesame seeds, and soybeans.[218]

When we eat properly, we can get almost all of the nutrients we need from food sources. However, Vitamin B-12 is only found in animal products, so most vegans and vegetarians take B-12 supplements. Sublingual liquid B vitamins with folic acid are more easily and quickly absorbed than pills. If you are concerned that you aren't getting sufficient vitamins in your diet and wish to take supplements, consult a holistic physician.

Chapter 11
Let's Eat

W e set out to write this book for a few reasons:
- We could not tolerate the cruelty associated with a meat-eating diet and we wanted to help end animal suffering.
- We couldn't bear to have "real" jobs.
- We wanted to change peoples' lives.

We *truly* want to help you succeed and make this all as easy as possible.

In this chapter, we've compiled a few lists so that there will be no confusion as to what you should or shouldn't eat. After reading the whole book, if you're feeling uncertain about what to buy or order, just whip out your little *Skinny Bitch* and come right to this chapter. There will be no doubt that you're making the right food choices.

Breakfast is the most important meal of the day. But not why you think. The cereal and dairy industries lead us to believe that without a big, "healthy" breakfast, we won't have enough energy to get us through the day. But Sugar Smacks with cow's milk hardly constitutes a healthy, viable energy source. The *real* reason breakfast is so important is that it sets the tone for your entire day of eating. If you eat a shitty breakfast, you will likely crave (and eat) crap all day. And, if you eat too early in the morning, you'll be interrupting your body's cleaning session. Remember, when your body isn't working on food, it's working on you! When your "cleaning crew" is in the middle of cleanup, and you start cramming food in, "they" get overwhelmed. They stop what they're doing, throw their hands up, scratch their heads, and finally, decide that they just can't deal with this mess you're making. So they opt to store it away as fat and pretend they'll get to it later.[219] So when you wake up, you should wait to eat breakfast until you're truly hungry. Don't just eat right away because that's what you're used to. After a few days, you'll grow to love that empty feeling in your stomach and know that the initial headaches, nausea, and hunger were just your body's cleaning crew. Feel free to enjoy a cup of caffeine-free, organic, herbal tea upon waking. But other than that, the best thing to do is wait until you're really hungry.

When you do eat, the breakfast of skinny bitches is organic fruit. This may seem light in comparison to your previous bagel or eggs or cereal. But again, once you adapt, you will be totally fulfilled by fruit. Eat one piece (or serving) slowly. After a period of time—perhaps ten minutes or so—when you feel hungry, eat another piece, slowly. When you feel hungry again, eat one more. Breakfast is over.

Breakfast Food List

We hope you'll at least try having just fruit for breakfast before deciding it's not for you. But if you give it a go, and after two weeks you still feel angry and violent just thinking about it, consult our list of acceptable breakfast foods:(R) found in refrigerator section, (F) found in freezer section

Arrowhead Mills: organic blue corn pancake and waffle mix

Arrowhead Mills: organic whole grain pancake and waffle mix

Food For Life: Ezekiel 4:9 cereal

Barbara's Bakery: Puffins cereal

Barbara's Bakery: Shredded Spoonfuls cereal

Peace Cereal: vanilla almond crisp

Peace Cereal: maple pecan crisp

Nature's Path: Optimum Slim cereal

Nature's Path: Optimum Power Breakfast cereal

Health Valley: organic raisin bran flakes

Health Valley: organic oat bran flakes with raisins

Old Wessex Ltd.: Irish-style oatmeal

Old Wessex Ltd.: 5-grain cereal

Nature's Path: organic instant hot maple nut oatmeal

Ancient Harvest: organic quinoa flakes

Rice Dream: original enriched rice milk

Original EdenSoy: organic soymilk

Original EdenBlend: rice & soy beverage

House: tofu steak (R)

Whole Soy & Co.: creamy cultured soy (yogurt) (R)

Silk: cultured soy (yogurt) (R)

Amy's: organic tofu scramble (F)

Van's: all natural organic original waffles (F)

Lifestream: Mesa Sunrise toaster waffles (F)

French Meadow Bakery: men's bread

French Meadow Bakery: healthy hemp sprouted bread

French Meadow Bakery: brown rice bread

Nature's Path: organic Manna breads (F)

Fabe's All Natural Bakery: vegan muffins (F)

Zen Bakery: muffins (R)

Zen Bakery: cinnamon raisin rolls (R)

Whole Foods: organic English muffins (R)

Food For Life: Ezekiel 4:9 sprouted grain bagels (F)

Tofutti: Better Than Cream Cheese (R) (the kind *without* hydrogenated oils.)

Lightlife: Smart Bacon (R)

Lightlife: Gimme Lean! sausage style (R)

Organic Fruit: (Earlier, we mentioned the benefit of eating just
fruit for breakfast. But here, we did include other breakfast foods.

It is up to you to decide how diligent you want to be with your diet. We just wanted to provide hearty breakfast choices should you disregard the fruit-by-itself theory. Totally your choice. You can eat the fruit before eating the muffin or pancakes or waffles. Whatever you want.)

Lunch Food List

Don't eat lunch until you're close to ravenous. This will allow your breakfast to pass through your body without having food piled on top of it. In a perfect, skinny world, lunch consists of a fresh, organic salad with lots of raw vegetables. But if that's too boring or stringent for you, feel free to choose something else from our yummy lunch list:

Food For Life: Ezekiel 4:9 bread (F) (or bakery/bread aisle)

Arrowhead Mills: organic Valencia peanut butter

MaraNatha: organic raw almond butter

I.M. Healthy: SoyNut butter

Bionaturae: organic fruit spreads

Natural Touch: Tuno (faux tuna)

Morningstar Farms: Tuno

Amy's: All American burger (F)

Amy's: California burger (F)

Amy's: Texas burger (F)

Gardenburger's: flame-grilled burgers (F)

Gardenburger's: flame-grilled chik'n (F)

Whole Foods Bakehouse: organic burger buns

Tofurkey: deli slices

Yves: veggie bologna (R)

Yves: veggie turkey (R)

Yves: veggie salami (R)

Follow Your Heart: Vegan Gourmet cheese alternative (R)

Earthbound Farm: organic salad greens (R)

Fantastic Foods: tabouli

Fantastic Foods: organic whole wheat couscous

Fantastic Carb 'Tastic Soup: vegetarian chicken gumbo

Fantastic Carb 'Tastic Soup: shiitake mushroom

Fantastic Big Soup: five bean

Fantastic Big Soup: country lentil

Amy's Organic Soups: black bean vegetable

Amy's Organic Soups: butternut squash

Amy's Organic Soups: lentil vegetable

Amy's Organic Soups: chunky vegetable

Amy's: organic chili

Health Valley: organic split pea soup

Health Valley: organic lentil soup

Health Valley: organic black bean soup

Imagine: organic vegetable broth

Imagine: organic no-chicken broth

Pacific: organic vegetable broth

organic vegetables

Dinner Food List

When you're feeling really hungry, it's time for din-din. Dinner is easy and fun. Just pick from the list, or create your own healthy vegan fest:

Health Best 100% Organic: red lentils

Health Best 100% Organic: green lentils

Health Best 100% Organic: barley

Health Best 100% Organic: split peas

Health Best 100% Organic: amaranth

Arrowhead Mills: organic whole millet

Lundberg Family Farms: organic short grain brown rice

Lundberg Family Farms: organic brown rice pasta

DeBoles: organic whole wheat pasta

Ancient Harvest: organic quinoa supergrain pasta

Eddie's Spaghetti: organic vegetable pasta

Pastariso: organic brown rice fettuccine

Pastariso: organic brown rice elbow macaroni

Rising Moon Organics: spinach Florentine ravioli with tofu (F)

Chef Nikola's Kitchen: roasted eggplant in herbed balsamic sauce (F)

Amy's Organic: Asian noodle stir-fry (F)

Amy's Organic: Thai stir-fry (F)

Amy's: roasted vegetable pizza (no cheese) (F)

Nate's: meatless meatballs (F)

Health is Wealth: buffalo wings (F)

Health is Wealth: chicken-free patties (F)

Health is Wealth: chicken-free nuggets (F)

Tofurkey: *Tofurkey* dinner (F)

Gloria's Kitchen: assorted vegan prepared entrees (F)

Lightlife: organic tempeh (R)

Lightlife: *Smart Ground* (ground "meat") (F)

Nasoya: organic tofu (R)

White Wave: chicken-style seitan (R)

Lightlife: *Smart Dogs* (R)

Yves: veggie dogs (R)

Rudi's Organic Bakery: white hot dog rolls

Now & Zen: *UnChicken* (R)

Now & Zen: *UnSteak* (R)

Yves: *Veggie Ground Round Mexican* (Mexican-style ground
    "meat") (F)

Bearitos: taco shells

Garden of Eatin': blue corn taco shells

Alvarado St. Bakery: organic sprouted wheat tortillas

organic vegetables

Obviously, the foods on the lunch and dinner lists can be used interchangeably.

A helpful hint: Prepare large batches of staple food items on

Sunday night, to tide you over for your busy workweek. Brown rice, lentils, homemade hummus, soups, and pastas are all good candidates. But try not to do this with your veggies because they'll lose some of their enzymatic punch.

Acceptable Junk Food, Snacks & Desserts

There's something about a snack that makes you feel like a kid again. And that's a good thing. If you're hungry, but not quite ready for dinner, have a small snack. As long as it's healthy, it doesn't spoil your dinner, and you only have a small serving, there is no reason to feel bad about having a snickety-snack. But don't have one just because you can. Only eat it if you want it. Otherwise, just wait for dinner.

Dessert is one of God's many gifts to humans. Indulge. Like snacks, if your desserts are healthy and eaten in controlled portions, enjoy them without the guilt!

365: organic chocolate soymilk

Whole Foods: organic date coconut rolls

Barbara's Bakery: organic graham crackers

Dagoba: organic dark chocolate bars

Uncle Eddie's: vegan cookies

Organica Foods: vegan cookies

Fabe's All Natural Bakery: vegan cookies

Newman's Own: organic Fig Newmans

Laura's Wholesome Junk Food: *Bitelettes* (cookies)

Nutrilicious Natural Bakery: donut holes

MI-DEL: vanilla snaps

Country Choice: certified organic sandwich cremes

Back to Nature: classic creme sandwich cookies

Back to Nature: chocolate & mint creme sandwich cookies

Chocolove: Belgian dark chocolate

Endangered Species: dark chocolate bars

Tropical Source: rice crisp dark chocolate

Ecco Bella: *Health By Chocolate*

Raw Balance: *Carobelles* (www.rawbalance.com)

Gertrude & Bronner's Magic: *Alpsnack*

LäraBar: all flavors

Terra: exotic vegetable chips original

Terra: spiced sweet potato chips

Maine Coast Sea Vegetables: sea chips

Garden of Eatin': *Sunny Blues* (tortilla chips with sunflower seeds)

Guiltless Gourmet: yellow corn baked chips

Kettle Organic Tortilla Chips: sesame blue moons

Veggie Stix: shoestring potato sticks

Robert's American Gourmet: *Tings*

Robert's American Gourmet: *Spicy Tings*

Robert's American Gourmet: *Veggie Booty*

Newman's Own: organic salted round pretzels

Koyo Organic Rice Cakes: dulse

Koyo Organic Rice Cakes: mixed grain

Nature's Path: tamari flax crackers

Back to Nature: classic rounds

Soy Dream: non-dairy frozen desserts (F)

Soy Delicious: non-dairy frozen desserts (F)

Double Rainbow Soy Cream: non-dairy desserts (F)

Soy Delicious: *Li'l Buddies* ("ice cream" sandwiches) (F)

Sweet Nothings: non-dairy fudge bars (F)

Condiments, Baking Supplies & Miscellaneous

Don't worry about the little odds and ends. We've thought of everything.

Earth Balance: natural buttery spread (R)

Soy Garden: natural buttery spread (R)

Follow Your Heart: *Vegenaise* (mayonnaise substitute) (R)

Nasoya: *Nayonaise*

Muir Glen: organic ketchup

Westbrae: natural ketchup

Whole Kids: organic yellow mustard

Spectrum Naturals: organic sesame oil

Spectrum Naturals: organic canola oil

Spectrum Naturals: organic extra virgin olive oil

MaraNatha: organic raw tahini

Bragg Liquid Aminos: all purpose seasoning (soy sauce substitute)

Sea Seasonings: organic kelp granules with cayenne

Annie's Naturals: goddess dressing

OrganicVille: sesame tamari organic vinaigrette

The Wizard's: organic original vegetarian Worcestershire sauce

Essential Living Foods: organic agave nectar or syrup

Shady Maple Farms: certified organic pure maple syrup

Sugar in the Raw: Turbinado sugar from natural cane

Florida Crystals: organic cane sugar

Wholesome Sweeteners: organic sucanat

Hain Pure Foods: organic brown sugar

Stevita Company Inc.: stevia spoonable

Dr. Oetker Organics: chocolate cake mix

Dr. Oetker Organics: vanilla cake mix

Dr. Oetker Organics: chocolate icing mix

Dr. Oetker Organics: vanilla icing mix

Dr. Oetker Organics: chocolate chip cookie mix

Ener-G: egg replacer

Chatfield's Carob & Compliments: dairy-free carob morsels

Sunspire: grain-sweetened chocolate chips

Arrowhead Mills: organic oat flour

Arrowhead Mills: organic whole wheat flour

Arrowhead Mills: organic spelt flour

Arrowhead Mills: organic brown rice flour

Arrowhead Mills: organic blue corn meal

Arrowhead Mills: organic yellow corn meal

Arrowhead Mills: organic flax seeds

When crafting your own day of eating from the food lists provided, use your head. Create a well-balanced menu for the day without being repetitive. For example, don't eat pancakes for breakfast, a sandwich for lunch, and a soy burger for dinner. That would be eating all bread, but no fruits or veggies. Duh. Use your head. Try to always think in terms of fruits, veggies, whole grains, soy, and legumes for a well-balanced day of eating.

If you need a little more guidance, feast your eyes on this, a month's worth of menus:

Week One

Monday

Breakfast: Mango, banana, kiwi and soy yogurt.

Lunch: Spinach salad with shredded carrots, chopped almonds, red onion, fresh garlic, cubed tofu, and sesame oil.

Dinner: Pasta with zucchini, tomatoes, garlic, fresh parsley, pine nuts, and olive oil.

Tuesday

Breakfast: Fresh squeezed orange juice, whole grain muffin with soy butter, banana, and strawberries.

Lunch: Tabouli salad with marinated tofu, eggplant, and red peppers.

Dinner: Veggie nachos! Corn chips with veggie chili, soy cheese, guacamole, scallions, and tomatoes.

Wednesday

Breakfast: Fresh squeezed grapefruit juice and slow-cooking oatmeal with blueberries, strawberries, and raspberries.

Lunch: Veggie burger on whole grain bun with red onion, lettuce, tomato, avocado, and alfalfa sprouts. Served with vegan potato salad.

Dinner: Fake chicken patty with brown rice, lentils, and steamed kale.

Thursday

Breakfast: Fresh squeezed OJ, whole grain bagel with vegan cream cheese, sliced tomatoes, and red onion.

Lunch: Soup and salad.

Dinner: Veggie stir-fry with peppers, onions, garlic, carrots, bok choy, and mushrooms served with brown rice and tofu.

Friday

Breakfast: Granola with sliced banana, peaches, and blueberries with soy yogurt.

Lunch: Club sandwich with fake bacon, fake turkey slices, avocado, lettuce, tomato, sprouts, and Vegenaise (fake mayo). Served with three-bean salad.

Dinner: Take out from your favorite Thai restaurant: vegan Pad Thai, emphasizing no egg or shrimp or fish stock.

Saturday

Breakfast: Fresh squeezed OJ, blue corn and blueberry pancakes served with fresh strawberries.

Lunch: Salad with shredded carrots, couscous, cranberries, and walnuts, dressed with citrus vinaigrette. Served with lentil soup.

Dinner: Veggie fajitas with sautéed peppers, onions, mushrooms, and fake chicken strips, topped with fresh Pico de Gallo.

Sunday

Breakfast: Fresh squeezed OJ and tofu scramble with zucchini, peppers, onions, garlic, spinach, and kale served with whole grain toast.

Lunch: Lentil salad with asparagus tips and walnuts in a raspberry vinaigrette. Served with an entire steamed artichoke and a vegan lemon-butter dipping sauce.

Dinner: No-cheese or vegan-cheese pizza loaded with veggies!

Week Two

Monday

Breakfast: Fruit smoothie with a splash of OJ and fresh banana, frozen pineapple, and coconut.

Lunch: All-American salad with romaine lettuce, corn, peas, and BBQ tofu cubes in a vegan ranch dressing.

Dinner: Italian night! Your favorite pasta and tomato sauce with fake meatballs and whole grain garlic bread.

Tuesday

Breakfast: Fresh squeezed OJ, cereal with soy or rice milk, served with blueberries, sliced banana, and strawberries.

Lunch: Veggie chili with corn bread!

Dinner: Mashed potatoes, Gardenburger Meatless Riblets, and
sautéed collard greens and Swiss chard.

Wednesday

Breakfast: Fresh squeezed OJ and toaster waffles with sliced strawberries, bananas, and peaches.

Lunch: Vegan Caesar salad with fake chicken chunks.

Dinner: Brown rice and lentils with steamed broccoli and red cabbage.

Thursday

Breakfast: A shitload of cantaloupe.

Lunch: Fake deli meats on whole grain bread with lettuce and tomato
and a side of Asian cole slaw (shredded carrots, red cabbage,
green cabbage, rice vinegar, sesame oil, and sesame seeds).

Dinner: Fake meatloaf served with corn on the cob, peas, and
sautéed spinach and garlic.

Friday

Breakfast: Smoothie time with a splash of apple juice and peaches,
blueberries, raspberries, and a dash of flaxseed oil (or a

tablespoon of ground flaxseeds).

Lunch: Japanese lunch of avocado rolls, miso soup, and a small salad.

Dinner: Veggie burger with sautéed mushrooms, onions, soy cheese, lettuce, and tomato served with baked French "fries."

Saturday

Breakfast: Fresh squeezed OJ and vegan French toast with blueberries, strawberries, and banana.

Lunch: Mixed greens with hearts of palm, sun-dried tomatoes, yellow tomatoes, asparagus, basil, garlic, and pine nuts in an oil and vinegar dressing.

Dinner: Veggie dog loaded with veggie chili and soy cheese, served with vegan potato salad.

Sunday

Breakfast: Fresh squeezed OJ and a fake egg sandwich (using House Tofu Steak extra-firm tofu, sliced and pan fried, with fake bacon and soy cheese on a whole grain bagel with soy butter, salt, pepper, and ketchup).

Lunch: Split pea soup and a mixed greens salad.

Dinner: Penne with butternut squash and raw pesto (pine nuts, basil, garlic, olive oil).

Week Three

Monday

Breakfast: Fresh squeezed OJ and slow-cooking oatmeal with apples, cinnamon, and pecans.

Lunch: Whole-wheat vegetable wrap with sautéed eggplant, portabella mushroom, and roasted red peppers served with a small side salad.

Dinner: Veggie stir-fry with green peppers, carrots, zucchini, tofu, bok choy, onions, and garlic served with brown rice.

Tuesday

Breakfast: A big-ass hunk of honeydew melon.

Lunch: Salad greens with red onion, cherry tomatoes, black beans, and corn, served with a baked sweet potato.

Dinner: Baked Teriyaki tofu with brown jasmine rice and steamed green beans.

Wednesday

Breakfast: Fresh- pressed apple juice and a whole grain bagel with peanut butter, jelly (organic and sugar-free, of course), and sliced banana.

Lunch: Mediterranean platter with hummus, eggplant, grape
leaves, falafel, peppers, olives, and tomatoes.

Dinner: Veggie burrito with pinto beans, brown rice, guacamole, soy
cheese, lettuce, tomato, and salsa.

Thursday

Breakfast: Granola with bananas, blueberries, strawberries, and
soy or rice milk.

Lunch: Portabella mushroom burger with arugula and caramelized
onions, served with an avocado-tomato salad.

Dinner: Veggie lasagna with red sauce, your favorite veggies, fake
ground meat, and tofu ricotta (in food processor, blend firm
tofu, garlic, salt, small amount of olive oil, and dried
oregano).

Friday

Breakfast: Fruit salad—go crazy!

Lunch: Fake tuna (Tuno with accents of shredded carrots, chopped
onion, diced celery, and Vegenaise) on whole grain bread
served with a handful of baked corn chips.

Dinner: Steamed broccoli, carrots, kale, red cabbage, cauliflower,
and tofu with brown rice, drizzled with sesame oil and sea salt.

Saturday

Breakfast: Ranchos-fake-Huevos wrap with scrambled tofu, sautéed onions and peppers, black beans, avocado, and salsa in a corn tortilla.

Lunch: Chinese fake chicken salad with snow peas, cabbage, carrots, mandarin oranges, fake chicken chunks, and cashews.

Dinner: Seitan (wheat-meat) with steamed leeks, white beans, and garlic-roasted potatoes.

Sunday

Breakfast: Fresh squeezed OJ and apple cinnamon pancakes with raspberries and bananas.

Lunch: Fake bacon, lettuce, tomato, and avocado on whole grain bread with leftover roasted potatoes from last night's dinner.

Dinner: Veggie shish kabobs with green peppers, red peppers, mushrooms, onions, cherry tomatoes, and Gardenburger Meatless Riblets, served with corn on the cob.

Week Four

Monday

Breakfast: Fruit smoothie with peaches, banana, and strawberries and a splash of soy or rice milk.

Lunch: Chef's salad with mixed greens, carrots, tomatoes, vegan cheese, and assorted chopped fake deli meats.

Dinner: Fake steak with a baked sweet potato, lentils, and steamed kale.

Tuesday

Breakfast: Fresh-squeezed OJ and toaster waffles with banana, strawberries, and blueberries.

Lunch: Veggie minestrone soup with a small side salad.

Dinner: Veggie dog smothered in veggie chili, served with collard greens.

Wednesday

Breakfast: Fresh-pressed apple juice and slow-cooked oatmeal with dates, raisins, walnuts, and bananas.

Lunch: Grilled soy cheese with tomato and a small side salad.

Dinner: Shepherd's pie with vegan mashed potatoes, fake ground meat, lentils, corn, and sautèed spinach and mushrooms.

Thursday

Breakfast: Fresh-squeezed OJ, an entire grapefruit, and a whole grain muffin.

Lunch: Veggie chili with an avocado-tomato salad and a handful of baked corn chips.

Dinner: Fusilli with zucchini, olives, basil, tomato, garlic, and olive oil served with whole grain Italian bread.

Friday

Breakfast: Fresh-squeezed OJ and cereal with peaches, banana, blackberries, and soymilk.

Lunch: Cucumber and avocado roll with miso soup and a small salad.

Dinner: No-cheese or vegan-cheese pizza loaded with veggies!

Saturday

Breakfast: Fake egg sandwich.

Lunch: Fake chicken Caesar salad.

Dinner: Steamed cauliflower, broccoli, carrots, and red cabbage over brown rice.

Sunday

Breakfast: Create your own fruit smoothie!

Lunch: Veggie burger with sautèed mushrooms, avocado, lettuce, tomato, onion, and sprouts served with roasted potato wedges.

Dinner: Fake chicken patty with BBQ sauce, black-eyed peas, collard greens, and corn on the cob.

*Feel free to snack on a handful of raw organic nuts each day.

**If you really want to treat yourself right, have fresh-pressed veggie juice every day. (Fresh-pressed, not packaged or pasteurized.)

***Don't forget to include organic, caffeine-free teas and to drink eight glasses of water a day.

****We include a list of recommended cookbooks toward the end of the book. Either buy a book or use the Internet for easy vegan recipes. One great site, veganpeace.com, includes recipes and a review of veggie cookbooks. Another winner is VegCooking.com.

Feeling gutsy and wanna branch out on your own? Go for it—shop 'till you drop. Here are ingredient lists of unfamiliar terms to help with your grocery outings. (Please be warned, this section is boring.)

Bad or Potentially
Bad Ingredients*

Alanine or amino acids: The building blocks of protein in all animals and plants. Make sure they are plant derived.

Albumen or albumin: Found in eggs, milk, muscles, blood, and many vegetable tissues and fluids. May cause allergic reaction. In cakes, cookies, candies, and some wines.

Ambergris: From whale intestines. Used as a flavoring in foods and beverages.

Aminosuccinate Acid or **aspartic acid:** Can be animal or plant source (e.g., molasses).

Arachidyl proprionate: A wax that can be from animal fat. Alternatives are peanut or vegetable oil.

Artificial Color, FD & C food color: Derived from coal-tar. Can contain trace amounts of lead and arsenic. Potentially carcinogenic. Alternatives: coloring from grapes, beets, turmeric, saffron, carrots, chlorophyll, annatto, alkanet.

Beta carotene, provitamin A: A pigment found in many animal tissues and in all plants. Used in the manufacturing of

Vitamin A. Make sure it is derived from plant sources.

Bone meal: Crushed or ground animal bones. In some vitamins and supplements as a source of calcium.

Butylated Hhydroxyanisole (BHA), butylated hydroxytoluene (BHT): An antioxidant and/or preservative commonly found in baked goods, canned items, powdered soups, bacon, foods containing artificial colors or flavors. Can cause cancer, birth defects, and infertility.

Carmine, cochineal, carminic acid: Red pigment from the crushed female cochineal insect. Reportedly, 70,000 beetles must be killed to produce one pound of this red dye. Used in red applesauce, and other foods (including red lollipops and food coloring). May cause allergic reaction.

Casein, caseinate, sodium caseinate: Milk protein found in dairy products, as well as "non-dairy" creamers, and soy cheese.

Cysteine, L-form: An amino acid from hair, which can come from animals. Used in some bakery products.

Cystine: An amino acid found in urine and horsehair. Used as a nutritional supplement.

Duodenum substances: From the digestive tracts of cows and pigs.

Added to some vitamin tablets.

Fatty acids: Can be one or any mixture of liquid and solid acids such as caprylic, lauric, myristic, oleic, palmitic, and stearic. Alternatives: vegetable-derived acids, soy lecithin.

Fish liver oil: Used in vitamins, supplements, and milk fortified with vitamin D. Alternative: yeast extract ergosterol.

Gelatin, gel: Protein obtained by boiling skin, tendons, ligaments, and/or bones with water. From cows and pigs. Used as a thickener for fruit gelatins and puddings and in vitamins as a coating and as capsules. In candies, marshmallows, cakes, ice cream, yogurts. Sometimes used to assist in "clearing" wines. Alternatives: carrageen (carrageenan, Irish moss), seaweeds (algin, agar-agar, kelp), pectin from fruits, dextrins, locust bean gum, cotton gum.

Glycerin, glycerol: A byproduct of soap manufacturing (normally uses animal fat). In foods, mouthwashes, chewing gum, toothpastes. Derivatives: Glycerides, Glyceryls, Glycrethglyceth-26, Polyglycerol. Alternatives: vegetable glycerin—a byproduct of vegetable oil soap, derivatives of seaweed.

Isinglass: A form of gelatin prepared from the internal membranes of fish bladders. Sometimes used in "clearing" wines and in foods. Alternatives: bentonite clay, "Japanese isinglass," agar-agar. (See alternatives to Gelatin).

Lactic acid: Found in blood and muscle tissue. Also in sour milk, beer, sauerkraut, pickles, and other food products made by bacterial fermentation. Alternative: lactic acid from beets, plant-milk sugars.

Lactose: Milk sugar from milk of mammals. In foods, tablets, baked goods. Alternatives: plant-milk sugars.

Lard: Fat from hog abdomens. In baked goods, French fries, refried beans. Alternatives: pure vegetable fats or oils.

Lecithin or choline bitartrate: Waxy substance in nervous tissue of all living organisms, but frequently obtained for commercial purposes from eggs and soybeans. Also from blood or milk. Alternatives: soybean lecithin or corn-derived.

Lipase: Enzyme from the stomachs and tongue glands of calves, baby goats, and lambs. Used in cheese-making and in digestive aids. Alternatives: vegetable enzymes, castor beans.

Lipoids, lipids: Fat and fat-like substances that are found in animals and plants. Alternatives: vegetable oils.

Marine oil: From fish or marine mammals (including porpoises). Used as a shortening, especially in some margarines. Alternatives: vegetable oils.

Methionine: Essential amino acid found in various proteins (usually from egg albumen and casein). Used for freshness in potato chips.

Monoglycerides, glycerides, (See Glycerin): From animal fat. In margarines, cake mixes, candies, foods, etc. Alternative: vegetable glycerides.

Monosodium glutamate (MSG): Flavor enhancer blamed for reproductive, nervous system, and brain disorders. Found in soups, sauces, gravies, and sometimes hidden in baby food, baby formula, low-fat and no-fat milk, candy, gum, processed foods, and applied to non-organic fruits and vegetables as a wax or pesticide.

Myristal, ether sulfate, myristic acid: Organic acid in most animal and vegetable fats. In butter acids and food flavorings. Derivatives: isopropyl myristate, myristal ether sulfate, myristyls, oleyl myristate. Alternatives: nut butters, oil of lovage, coconut oil, extract from seed kernels of nutmeg, etc.

"Natural sources": Can mean animal or vegetable sources. Most often in the health food industry (especially in the cosmetics area), it means animal sources, such as animal elastin, glands, fat, protein, and oil. Alternatives: plant sources.

Nitrates: Potentially deadly, carcinogenic preservatives. Found in processed foods and meats.

Nucleic acids: In the nucleus of all living cells. Used in vitamins, supplements. Alternatives: plant sources.

Oleic acid: Obtained from various animal and vegetable fats and oils. Usually obtained commercially from inedible tallow. (See Tallow.) Alternatives: coconut oil.

Olestra: A fat substitute found in low fat and dairy-type products that reduces fat-soluble vitamins in the body.

Panthenol, dexpanthenol, vitamin B-Complex complex factor, provitamin B-5: Can come from animal, plant, or synthetic sources, so be sure to buy only plant-based.

Pepsin: In hogs' stomachs. A clotting agent. In some cheeses and vitamins. Same uses and alternatives as Rennet. (see Rennet)

Polysorbates: Derivatives of fatty acids.

Potassium bisulfite, sodium bisulfite, sulfur dioxide: Used as anti-fungal, anti-browning, or antioxidant in cheeses, processed meats, canned fruits and vegetables, dried fruits, and/or baked goods. Can cause asthma, shock, or death.

Potassium bromate: Found in baked goods, can cause cancer and kidney and nervous system disorders. Banned worldwide except Japan and U.S.

Rapeseed Oil: An emulsifier and stabilizer found in baked goods, dairy products, processed meats. Can cause cancer, heart disease, vision loss.

Rennet, rennin: Enzyme from calves' stomachs. Used in cheese-making and in many coagulated dairy products. Alternatives: lemon juice or vegetable rennet.

Saccharine: Artificial sweetener found to cause cancer.

Stearic acid: Fat from cows and sheep and from dogs and cats euthanized in animal shelters, etc. Most often refers to a fatty substance taken from the stomachs of pigs. Used in gum, food flavoring. Derivatives: stearamide, stearamine, stearates, stearic hydrazide, stearone, stearoxytrimethylsi-lane, stearoyl lactylic acid, stearyl betaine, stearyl imidazoline. Alternatives: Stearic acid can be found in many vegetable fats, coconut.

Tallow, fatty alcohol: Rendered beef fat. May cause eczema and blackheads.

Urea, uric acid, carbamide: Excreted from urine and other bodily fluids. Used to "brown" baked goods, such as pretzels. Derivatives: imidazolidinyl urea, uric acid.

Vitamin A: Can come from fish liver oil (e.g., shark liver oil), egg yolk, butter, and synthetics. In vitamins, supplements. Alternatives: carrots, other vegetables, lemongrass, wheat germ oil.

Vitamin B-12: Can come from animal products or bacteria cultures. Alternatives: Vegetarian vitamins, fortified soymilks, nutritional yeast, fortified faux meat substitutes. Vitamin B-12 is often listed as "cyanocobalamin" on food labels. Vegan health professionals caution that vegans get 5-10 mcg/day of vitamin B-12 from fortified foods or supplements .

Vitamin D, ergocalciferol, vitamin D-2, ergosterol, provitamin D-2, calciferol, vitamin D-3: Vitamin D can come from fish liver oil, milk, egg yolk, etc. Vitamin D-2 can come from animal fats or plant sterols. Vitamin D-3 is always from an animal source. Alternatives: plant and mineral sources, completely vegetarian vitamins, exposure of skin to sunlight.

Whey: A derivative of milk. Usually in cakes, cookies, candies, and breads. Used in cheese-making. Alternatives: soybean whey.

Bear in mind, even though these are on our "bad" list, they are fine when derived from non-chemical, non-animal sources.

Scary-Sounding But Actually Harmless Ingredients*

Alpha tocopherol, Alpha tocopherol acetate: Vitamin E derived from corn, peanuts, or soy.

Arrowroot: A natural thickening starch, derived from the arrowroot plant.

Absorbic acid: Synthetic vitamin C, often derived from corn.

Brown rice syrup: A sweetener derived from brown rice.

Cellulose: Plant fiber.

Coconut Oil: Great for frying and baking because it can withstand high heats without becoming carcinogenic. Also helps the body metabolize fatty acids.

Date Sugar: Sweetener derived from dates.

Inulin: Present in many herbs. Acts as a probiotic and promotes healthy intestinal tract.

Linoleic acid: Derived from corn, soy, or peanuts.

Saffron: Natural food coloring derived from a plant.

Sucanat: SUgar CAne NATural, a natural sweetener.

*Sourced from *Food Additives: A Shopper's Guide To What's Safe & What's Not* by Christine Hoza Farlow, D.C., and PETA's *Caring Consumer Guide.*[220]

Chapter 12
FYI

U m, just bcause we wrote this book doesn't mean we're perfect. If you see us eating junk food or doing beer bongs, don't hold it against us. We believe in enjoying life *and* maintaining a healthy balance. We're human. Also, we have some fat, gross body parts, too. We're women.

❧

Yeah, eating onions and garlic makes your breath smell like someone took a shit down your throat. But they fight cancer and help detoxify your liver. So eat 'em.

◆

What's all the drama surrounding hydrogenated oils? We'll tell you. Manufacturers add hydrogen to mono- or polyunsaturated fats (good fats), in order to change their consistencies. The end result, trans-fatty acids (bad), is a more solid product with a longer shelf life. Margarines, cookies, cakes, doughnuts, potato chips, meat and dairy products, and shortening can all contain hydrogenated oils. Trans-fatty acids can cause derangements of cell structure, accelerated aging, and a predisposition to diseases.[221]

Think about it. They are literally altering a naturally occurring product's molecular structure by adding hydrogen molecules to it. Eating these chemically altered foods containing hydrogenated oils will increase your risk of heart disease. Sad to say, heating oil at high temperatures also changes its natural molecular configuration and produces free-radicals. Free-radicals not only destroy essential fats and vitamins but are also linked to cancer and heart disease.[222] This is why olive oil and peanut oil, which are both healthy, can be very *unhealthy* in dishes like fried eggplant or

French fries. Avoid eating fried foods (sniffle) and re-using heated oils. Never heat oil to the point where it is smoking. Cook with canola oil or coconut oil using low heat and for the shortest amount of time possible.

❧

Don't be a cheap asshole. Yeah, yeah, yeah, organic produce is usually more expensive than conventional produce. But we spend countless dollars on clothes, jewelry, manicures, magazines, rent or mortgages, car payments, and other bullshit. Surely our health and our bodies (we only get one body) are more important than anything else in our lives. Even if you are spending more on organic food, you'll save money in the long run if you're preparing more meals and snacks at home (which is always cheaper than buying food on the fly). Organic is worth the extra money, and you should aim to have everything you eat be organic. But especially when buying fruits or vegetables that you eat without peeling the skin. Always buy organic blueberries, strawberries, raspberries, apples, and pears. Peanuts and peanut butter, too, because conventional ones are loaded with pesticides. Buying organic produce is the only way to guarantee you're not eating genetically modified organisms. According to *Food Additives: A Shopper's Guide to What's Safe & What's Not,* "genes are taken from one species of plant, animal or virus and inserted into another species in order to produce a desirable trait, such as disease resistance or hardier crops. No one knows the long-term effects of eating genetically modified foods. Genetically modified foods are being sold now and they are not being labeled. Certified organic foods are the only foods guaranteed not to be genetically modified."[223]

❧

Brushing your teeth is a great way to ward off sweet cravings and stop yourself from eating. But, two or three times a day, every day for your entire life, you swallow trace amounts of toothpaste. What's in it? Chemicals? Artificial sweeteners? Would you eat it? Read the ingredients. Buy natural.

❧

The skin is the body's largest organ. Every day, we slop all sorts of potions and lotions and makeup on ourselves, and rub them into our skin. Ever read the ingredients of these products? Ever consider that you are putting chemicals directly onto your largest organ? Ever think about the pores all over your body and what you're putting inside them? Hopefully, you will now. Buy natural beauty products. What you put *on* your body is just as important as what you put *in* your body (because, in essence, what you put on your body will wind up in your body), especially on body parts you shave, pluck, or wax. Open pores do not want chemicals bulldozing through. Are your deodorant, makeup, perfumes, and lotions safe?

You can get too much of a good thing. So don't overdose on water, or you'll flush necessary salt supplies right out of your body. Eight glasses a day is a good target.

Natural, unrefined Celtic sea salt (different from table salt) contains many essential minerals, enhances organ function, and neutralizes toxins. It also contributes to the hydration of our cells and organs.[224]

❧

Buy a food steamer. It will change your life.

❧

Do yoga. It is a kick-ass cardio workout that will strengthen, tone, and harden your muscles. Yoga is amazing for organ function, immune system strength, tackling insomnia, improving PMS symptoms and menstrual cramps, and overall health. You will love how it makes you look and feel. All kidding aside, if everyone did yoga, we would have world peace.

❧

Donate blood. You can save a life and lose weight at the same time.

❧

Keep your eyes peeled for bad press regarding veganism. It's usually planted by the industries that are threatened by the movement. Don't believe any of it. It's all bogus bullshit. One study claimed that feeding children a vegan diet was tantamount to child abuse. It just so happens that the National Cattlemen's Beef Association paid for the study. They had the gall to experiment on African children who were literally starving. These children were eating nothing but corn and beans in minuscule servings. When servings of meat were added to their diets, their health improved.[225] Well, of course it did. They were fucking starving. This doesn't prove that veganism is dangerous or unhealthy. It just shows that the National Cattlemen's Beef Association will exploit starving, impoverished children to create bad press for veganism and boost its own meat sales. This is nothing short of a disgrace and an embarrassment to America.

Chapter 13

Use Your Head

on't be a fat pig anymore. You know what you have to do, now do it. But don't go anorexic on us, either. It's easy to get caught up in any lifestyle change and go overboard. Make healthy choices and take excellent care of yourself without getting neurotic and obsessive.

USE YOUR HEAD. We can't say it enough. Use your own head and think about what you are eating. Forget what you've ever read, heard, or learned and just think for yourself. Once they've recovered, your body, brain, and instincts will always lead you down the right food path. Obey them and disregard everyone and everything else. You know the truth.

Read the ingredients. This goes hand in hand with using your head. If you plan on eating something, you should know exactly what it is. Even if it's a product that we've recommended, you still need to check the ingredients. Companies change their recipes all the time. Two vegan products we loved initially and suggested weren't vegan by the time we were finished writing this book, and we had to remove them from our recommendation lists. Trust no one. Not even us. Some of the products on our suggested food lists aren't perfect; we make certain allowances based on our own opinions and desires. Read and decide for yourself. And if you don't recognize an ingredient, call the company's 800 number on the package and ask what it is. If it's not something you would put in your body, tell them, and suggest that they improve their product. Companies really do take comments into account, so always voice your opinion.

Now that you're a Skinny Bitch, don't turn into a skinny bitch. We conceived of the title, *Skinny Bitch*, to get attention and sell books. We just wanted to spread our message far and wide and thought *Skinny Bitch* was a good way to do it. But we are not bitches, and we have no desire to promote bitchiness. There is nothing uglier than a pretty woman who's nasty. If you look great, you should feel good about yourself and be happy. Instead of fixating on the last five pounds you want to lose, celebrate the five you already lost. Progress, not perfection. Don't be insecure or competitive or feel threatened by women who are thinner or prettier than you. Be happy for them; it will make you look better. Smile a lot, give compliments out whenever you can, and be nice to everyone. You'll just keep getting prettier and prettier and skinnier and skinnier.

Soon, you'll notice people (especially men) flocking to the new you. Not just because you're skinny but because you are happier, healthier, and eating a cruelty-free diet. So feel free to share your new wealth of information with everyone who asks. Spread the good word, but be careful not to preach. You'll see that some people get very defensive about their diets when you tell them about yours. Even if you are being very non-judgmental, people may feel threatened by your righteousness. Understandably, your being a vegan shines a spotlight on the cruelty they're contributing to, and it makes them feel uncomfortable. When asked, you can describe what you've learned about the treatment of farm animals and all of the health benefits of being vegan. By all means, let people know how great you feel and how much weight you've lost. But never suggest that they try it or make them feel bad about their diet. Offer to lend them your copy of *Skinny Bitch*, or give them the GoVeg.com website. But don't push it. Everyone seeks the truth in his or her own time.

Now that you've got your diet, health, and appearances under control, fix other areas of your life. After all, there's no point in being gorgeous if your life is a mess. End your co-dependent relationship, quit your dead-end job, and ditch your toxic friends. Make a list of goals and start chipping away at them. THIS IS YOUR LIFE! Live it to the fullest with reckless abandon. Seize the day. And do it again tomorrow. Live. Go get your dream job. Search for your dream man. Fear nothing. Try everything. Be excited. Dance. You'll never get yesterday back, but today is yours for the taking. Make it great.

Bravo. You've got your life and your diet on-track. But you still need to move your ass. Exercise will boost your self-esteem, reduce your junk-food cravings, and help you *lose weight*. If you can commit to a gym routine, fantastic! You will reach your fitness goals faster. But you don't need to be a gym rat. Just do something! It can even be fun. Take a class that you've always wondered about, like kickboxing or belly dancing. Go for walks after dinner or bike rides on weekends. Better yet, walk or bike to work. Whatever you choose, exercise makes you feel great about yourself. And that alone is priceless.

You *are* what you *think*. Our thoughts, feelings, beliefs, and experiences create tangible, concrete reactions at cellular and atomic levels. So whether something is "real" or not doesn't matter. If we think, feel, believe, or experience it, it will become a reality. Slow down and think about this and realize the implications it can have on your life. It can work for or against you. For example, if you *think* you are fat and that diets never work and that you'll always be fat, then yes, you *are* fat and diets never work and you will always be fat. What you *think* actually becomes embedded in your brain and your cells and the energy field surrounding you. Your thoughts are just that powerful. So if you *feel* you are meant to be thin, and *believe Skinny Bitch* will make you lose weight and *know* that this book is going to change your life, you *will* be thin, you *will* lose weight, and your life *will* change. It is just that simple.

In her book, *Anatomy of the Spirit*, Dr. Caroline Myss examines the unquestionable link between negative emotions and physical illnesses. Take "Julie," for example. Julie's husband treated her with contempt and disdain, frequently said the mere sight of her repulsed him, and refused to sleep with her. It is no coincidence that Julie was diagnosed with breast and ovarian cancer, reflecting her lack of self-love for her "womanhood." She could not leave her husband. She never recovered from her cancer and died as a result.[226] "Joanna" was married to a man who had multiple affairs, which she knew about but tried to live with. Not surprisingly, she developed breast cancer. Eventually, she confronted her husband and demanded fidelity. However, he was unable to change, so she left the marriage. Joanna recovered from her cancer. *Anatomy of the Spirit* chronicles one history after another of people sickening themselves or healing themselves with thought and emotion. (Of course, we are not suggesting that everyone suffering from a disease has brought it upon him or herself. We are, however, saying it is entirely possible to do so.)

Our minds are infinitely powerful. Our favorite self-help gurus, Dr. Wayne Dyer, Louise Hay, and Tony Robbins, understand this, and they all preach the power of daily affirmations. An affirmation is a positive statement you make that allows you to clearly envision a goal or mindset. It is declared as if it is already happening, and it can be anything you want:

"Every day in every way my ass is getting smaller."

"Every day in every way my thighs are getting thinner."

"Every day in every way my stomach is getting flatter."

"Every day in every way I'm losing more and more weight."

"Every day in every way I'm loving my body more."

"Every day in every way I'm getting healthier and healthier."

Create your own affirmations and say them (in your head or aloud, if you can) when you wake up in the morning, while exercising, in your car, and in bed at night. You will immediately notice how good they make you feel and you will be astonished at the results. This book is the result of our affirmations, so we *know* they truly work.

Now that you love yourself, wear sexy clothes. You worked hard for this body and you should be proud of it. We know it can be terrifying to wear something super-trendy—like you don't have the right or aren't worthy. But you *are* good enough, you *do* deserve it, and no one is thinking otherwise. So don't be afraid of wearing revealing, high-fashion clothes. This is your body for this lifetime. Dress it up and love it. Why are you "saving" all your good underwear or hot outfits? Wear them, fool. But please keep in mind that looking cheap or cheesy doesn't accomplish anything. If you have poor fashion sense (you know who you are), ask someone for guidance.

Now we know we keep encouraging you to look your best, but, for the love of God, don't associate your worth with your appearance. We are spiritual beings walking around in these crazy skin suits. Our insides are much more important than our outsides. So don't you fucking dare measure your worth by the amount of attention or validation you get from men. It's nice to be appreciated, but it is not a necessity. Love yourself and your looks, even if no one else seems to. In time, your confidence and self-love will attract a winner.

Well, it's all there in black and white. We sincerely hope you will take the knowledge you've learned and put it to use from this moment on. YOU hold the power to change your life, and it's really so simple. Use your head, lose your ass.

Afterword

Isn't man an amazing animal? He kills wildlife by the millions in order to protect his domestic animals and their feed. Then he kills domestic animals by the billions and eats them. This in turn kills man by the millions, because eating all those animals leads to degenerative—and fatal—health conditions like heart disease, kidney disease, and cancer. So then man tortures and kills millions more animals to look for cures for these diseases. Elsewhere, millions of other human beings are being killed by hunger and malnutrition because food they could eat is being used to fatten domestic animals. Meanwhile, some people are dying of sad laughter at the absurdity of man, who kills so easily and so violently, and once a year sends out cards praying for "Peace on Earth."

—Preface from *Old MacDonald's Factory Farm,*
by C. David Coates

Recommended Reading

Books

Slaughterhouse, Gail A. Eisnitz. *This book is an absolute *must-read* for every American who has ever eaten meat, is still considering eating meat, or isn't sure if they should or shouldn't. Buy this book today!

Vegan: The New Ethics of Eating, Erik Marcus

The Food Revolution, John Robbins

Fast Food Nation, Eric Schlosser

Breaking the Food Seduction, Neal Barnard, M.D.

Carbophobia: The Sorry Truth About America's Low-Carb Craze, Michael Greger, M.D.

A Way Out: Dis-ease Deception & The Truth About Health, Matthew Grace (matthewgrace.com)

Magazines

VegNews (vegnews.com)   *Satya* (satyamag.com)

Spiritual/Self-Help Books/CDs

Your Erroneous Zones, Dr. Wayne Dyer

Real Magic, Dr. Wayne Dyer

You'll See It When You Believe It, Dr. Wayne Dyer

Notes from a Friend, Anthony Robbins

Get the Edge CDs, Anthony Robbins

You Can Heal Your Life, Louise L. Hay

Anatomy of the Spirit, Caroline Myss, Ph.D.

Cookbooks

The Uncheese Cookbook, Joanne Stepaniak

The Garden of Vegan, Tanya Barnard and Sara Kramer

How it all Vegan, by Tanya Barnard and Sara Kramer

The Compassionate Cook, PETA & Ingrid Newkirk

CalciYum, David & Rachelle Bronfman

The Native Foods Restaurant Cookbook, Tanya Petrovna

The Candle Cafè Cookbook, Joy Pierson and Bart Potenza with
Barbara Scott-Goodman

Viva le Vegan!, Dreena Burton

Very Vegetarian, Jannequin Bennet

Veganpeace.com offers recipes and reviews of veggie cookbooks

Restaurant Guides

vegoutguide.com

happycow.net

vegdining.com

The Tofu Tollbooth, Elizabeth Zipern and Dar Williams

VegOut: Vegetarian Dining Guide to New York City,
    Justin Schwartz

VegOut: Vegetarian Dining Guide to Seattle and Portland,
    George B. Stevenson

VegOut: Vegetarian Dining Guide to Washington, D.C.,
    Andrew Evans

VegOut: Vegetarian Dining Guide to San Francisco,
    Michele Ana Jordan

VegOut: Vegetarian Dining Guide to Southern California,
    Kathy Lynn Siegel

VegOut: Vegetarian Dining Guide to Chicago,
    Margaret Littman

VegOut: Vegetarian Dining Guide to Houston,
    Ann Sieber

VegOut: Vegetarian Dining Guide to Salt Lake City/Denver,
    Andrea Mather

Merchandise
Web Sites

veganstore.com

VeganEssentials.com

AnimalRights Stuff.com

AlternativeOutfitters.com

feelgoodtees.com

mooshoes.com

veganunlimited.com

TheVegetarianSite.com

VegSexShop.com

Web Sites

skinnybitch.net

GoVeg.com

meat.org

peta.org

farmsanctuary.org

pcrm.org

cok.net

protectinganimals.org

veganmd.org

atkinsexposed.org

VeganOutreach.org

afa-online.org

informedeating.org

organicconsumers.org

holisticmed.com

congress.org

anthonyrobbinsdc.com

drwaynedyer.com

hayhouse.com

oa.org (overeaters anonymous), 505-891-2664

Food Web Sites

vegieworld.com

deliciouschoices.com

veganstore.com

rawbalance.com

playfood.org

TreeHugginTreats.com

simpletreats.com

chocolatedecadence.com

leaheyfoods.com

vegandreams.com

goodbaker.com

rosecitychocolates.com

eatraw.com

nutrilicious.com

allisonsgourmet.com

healthy-eating.com

Sources Consulted

Armstrong, Clare, MS, RD. DiscoveryHealth.com. The Discovery Channel, updated Sept. 25, 2002; accessed Jan. 20, 2005

http://health.discovery.com/encyclopedias/1940.html

Aspartame Victims Support Group, presidiotex.com, updated Jan. 13, 2005; accessed Jan. 20, 2005, http://www.presidiotex.com/aspartame/

Atkins, Robert C., M.D. *Dr. Atkins' New Diet Revolution.* New York: Avon, 2002.

Baillie-Hamilton, Paula, M.D., Ph.D. *The Body Restoration Plan.* New York: Avery, 2003.

"Banned as Human Food, StarLink Corn Found in Food Aid." *Environmental News Service,* Feb. 16, 2005; accessed Feb. 20, 2005, http://www.ens-newswire.com/ens/feb2005/2005-02-16-09.asp#anchor2

"Barcelona Report," presidiotex.com, Jan. 12, 2005, accessed Sept. 9, 2005, http://www.presidiotex.com/barcelona/

Barnard, Neal M.D. *Breaking The Food Seduction: The Hidden Reasons Behind Food Cravings—and 7 Steps to End Them Naturally.* New York: St. Martin's, 2003.

Beck, Leslie, R.D. *The Ultimate Nutrition Guide For Women: How to Stay Healthy with Diet, Vitamins, Minerals, and Herbs.* Hoboken: John Wiley & Sons, 2001.

Bellon, Roberta. National Justice League. "Aspartame Lawsuits Accuse Many Companies Of Poisoning The Public," April 6, 2004, accessed Feb. 10, 2005, http://www.newmediaexplor er.org/sepp/2004/04/09/aspar tame_neurotoxic_coca_cola_pepsi_nutra_sweet_sued_in_cali fornia.htm

Boschen, Hank. "Cycles of the Body," thejuiceguy.com, Feb. 10, 2005, http://www.juiceguy.com/cycle.shtml

Bray, George A., Samara Joy Nielson, and Barry M. Popkin. "Consumption of high-fructose corn syrup in beverages may play a role in the epidemic of obesity." *American Journal of Clinical Nutrition,* Vol. 79, No. 4, 537-543, April 2004, http://www.ajcn.org/cgi/content/abstract/79/4/537. 1 From the Pennington Biomedical Research Center, Louisiana State University, Baton Rouge, LA (GAB), and the Department of Nutrition, University of North Carolina, Chapel Hill (SJN and BMP).

Brown, Harold. e-mail to Rory Freedman, March 21, 2005.

Brownlee, Christen. *The Beef about UTIs,* Vol. 167 no. 3, Jan. 15, 2005; accessed Jan. 20, 2005, http://www.sciencenews.org/articles/20050115/food.asp

Burros, Marian. "Splenda's 'Sugar' Claim Unites Odd Couple of Nutrition Wars." *New York Times,* Feb. 15, 2005; accessed Feb. 20, 2005, www.skyhen.org/CorporatePower/splendas_

sugar_ claim_unites_odd_couple_of_nutrition_wars.php

Caffeine. eCureMe Inc., accessed Feb. 10, 2005,
http://life.ecureme.com/healthyliving/naturalmedicine/n_caff
eine.asp

Caring Consumer Guide. Peta.org, accessed March 26, 2005,
www.caringconsumer.com/ingredientslist.html

Chandel, Amar. "Sweet Poison," *The Tribune Spectrum,* March 14,
2004; accessed March 22, 2005, www.tribuneindia.com/2004/
20040314/spectrum/main1.htm

Cichoke, Anthony J., D.C. *Enzymes & Enzyme Therapy: How to
Jump Start Your Way to Lifelong Good Health.* New Canaan:
Keats Publishing Inc., 1994.

Coates, C. David. *Old MacDonald's Factory Farm.* New York: The
Continuum Publishing Co., 1989.

Cohen, Robert. *Essence of Betrayal,* accessed March 1, 2005,
http://www.notmilk.com/forum/594.html

"Common Dairy Digestive Under-Recognized and Under-
Diagnosed in Minorities." Johnson & Johnson, accessed Feb.
13, 2005, ww.jnj.com/news/jnj_news/20020311_0944.htm

Cook, Christopher D. "Environmental Hogwash: The EPA works
with factory farms to delay regulation of 'Extremely
Hazardous Substances.' " Oct. 6, 2004; accessed Jan. 27,
2005,
www.inthesetimes.com/site/main/print/environmental_hogwa

sh/

Cousens, Gabriel M.D. *Conscious Eating.* Berkeley: North Atlantic Books, 2000.

Cousin, Jean Pierre and Kirsten Hartvig. *Vitality Foods For Health and Fitness.* London: Duncan Baird, 2002.

Davis, Gail. "A Tale of Two Sweeteners: Aspartame & Stevia," accessed Feb. 12, 2005, http://suewidemark.netfirms.com/davis.htm

Des Maisons, Kathleen, Ph.D. *Potatoes Not Prozac.* New York: Fireside, 1998.

Diamond, Harvey and Marilyn. *Fit For Life.* New York: Warner, 1985.

Diamond, Harvey and Marilyn. *Fit For Life II: Living Health.* New York: Warner, 1987.

Eisnitz, Gail A. 'Ask the Experts.' Peta.org, accessed March 17, 2005, www.goveg.com/vegkit/meet.asp

Eisnitz, Gail A. *Slaughterhouse: The Shocking Story of Greed, Neglect, and Inhumane Treatment Inside the U.S. Meat Industry.* Amherst: Prometheus Books, 1997.

"Factory Farming: Environmental Consequences." Animalalliance.ca, accessed March 29, 2005, www.animalalliance.ca/kids/facfar1.htm#environment

"Fact vs. Fiction." Thetruthaboutsplenda.com, accessed Feb. 14, 2005, www.truthaboutsplenda.com/factvsfiction/index.html

Farlow, Christine Hoza, D.C. *Food Additives: A Shopper's Guide to What's Safe & What's Not*. Escondido: KISS for Health, 2004.

"FDA Approved Animal Drug Products." FDA 'Green Book' section, accessed March 21, 2005, http://dil.vetmed.vt.edu/NadaFirst/ NADA.cfm

"Fish and Shellfish: Contamination Problems Preclude Inclusion in the Dietary Guidelines for Americans." Pcrm.org, Spring 2004, accessed March 31, 2005, www.pcrm.org/health/reports/ fish_report.html

"Fish Feel Pain." Fishinghurts.com, accessed March 3, 2005, www.fishinghurts.com/FishFeelPain.asp

"Food Additives." New-fitness.com, accessed Feb. 4, 2005, www.new-fitness.com/nutrition/food_additives.html

"Food and Nutrition Assistance Programs." Economic Research Service, U.S. Department of Agriculture, USDA.gov; updated March 18, 2005; accessed March 22, 2005, www.ers.usda.gov/Briefing/FoodNutritionAssistance/

"Free-Range Eggs and Meat: Conning Consumers?" Peta.org, accessed March 16, 2005, http://www.peta.org/mc/factsheet_display.asp?ID=96

Fuhrman, Joel M.D. *Eat to Live*. Boston, New York, London: Little, Brown, 2003.

Gates, Donna. *The Body Ecology Diet.* (excerpt from), accessed Feb. 25, 2005, http://www.holisticmed.com/sweet/stv-cook.txt

Gee, Margaret. *Words of Wisdom Calendar*. Kansas City, MI: Andrews McMeel, 2004.

Gold, Mark. "Formaldehyde Poisoning from Aspartame," Dec. 9, 1998; accessed March 6, 2005, www.holisticmed.com/aspartame/embalm.html

Gold, Mark. "Aspartame/NutraSweet Toxicity Summary" Nov. 30, 2000; accessed March 3, 2005, www.holisticmed.com/aspartame/summary.html

Gold, Mark. "Common Toxic and Unhealthy Substances to Avoid," accessed Feb. 28, 2005, http://www.holisticmed.com/aspartame/history.faq

Gold, Mark. "Scientific Abuse in Methanol/Formaldehyde Research Related to Aspartame," accessed Jan. 12, 2005, http://www.holisticmed.com/aspartame/abuse/methanol.html

Gold, Mark. "Toxicity Effects of Aspartame Use," accessed Feb. 2, 2005, www.holisticmed.com/aspartame/

Gold, Mark D. "The Bitter Truth about Artificial Sweeteners." truthcampaign.ukf.net. accessed March 23, 2005, http://www.truthcampaign.ukf.net/ articles/health/aspartame.html

Grace, Matthew. *A Way Out: Dis-Ease Deception and The Truth About Health.* U.S.A: Matthew Grace, 2000.

"The Great Sugar Debate: Is It Vegan?" accessed Feb. 20, 2005, http://www.vegfamily.com/articles/sugar.htm

Greger, Michael, M.D. "Rocket Fuel in Milk," accessed Jan. 23,
    2005, http://all-creatures.org/health/rocket.html

Green, Che. "Not Milk: The USDA, Monsanto, and the U.S. Dairy
    Industry." *LiP Magazine,* July 9, 2002; accessed Feb. 20, 2005,
    http://www.alternet.org/story/13557/

Grogan, Bryanna Clark. "A Few Words About Sugar and Other
    Sweeteners," accessed Feb. 22, 2005,
    http://www.vegsource.com/articles/bryanna_sugar.htm

"Growing and Processing Sugar." The Sugar Association; accessed
    Jan. 12, 2005, http://www.sugar.org/facts/grow.html

Harris, Simon. "Organic Consumers Association (OCA)
    Denounces Degradation of Organic Food Standards by
    Congress,"accessed Feb. 10, 2005,
    http://environment.about.com/ library/pressrelease/bloca.htm

Hasselberger, Sepp. "Aspartame: RICO Complaint Filed Against
    NutraSweet, ADA, Monsanto." Sept. 17, 2004; accessed Feb.
    15, 2005, http://www.newmediaexplorer.org/sepp/2004/09/17/
    aspartame_rico_complaint_filed_against_nutrasweet_ada_m
    onsanto.htm

Hatherill, Robert J., Ph.D. *Eat to Beat Cancer.* Los Angeles:
    Renaissance Books, 1998.

Healthy Child Online Articles and Resources, accessed March 2,
    2005, http://www.healthychild.com/database/life_is_sweet_
    a_guide_to_using_healthy_sweeteners.htm

"The Hidden Lives of Chickens," accessed March 3, 2005,

http://www.peta.org/feat/hiddenlives/

Holford, Patrick. *The Optimum Nutrition Bible.* Berkeley: The
    Crossing Press, 1999.

Howell, Edward M.D. *Enzyme Nutrition: The Food Enzyme
    Concept.* U.S.A.: Avery, 1985.

Howell, Laurie. "#193 Why Choose Organic Coffee?" accessed
    Feb. 25, 2005, http://www.thegreenscene.com/shows/193.html

"Investigation Reveals Slaughter Horrors at Agriprocessors."
    Peta.org, accessed March 17, 2005, www.goveg.com/feat/
    agriprocessors/

Johnson, Lucy. "Aspartame . . . A Killer!" *The Sunday Express*
    London, U.K. Newfrontier.com; accessed March 21, 2005,
    http://www.newfrontier.com/asheville/aspartame.htm

Kamen, Betty, Ph.D. *New Facts About Fiber*. Novato: Nutrition
    Encounter, 1991.

Krebs, A.V. "USDA Accused of Allowing 'Sham Certifiers' into the
    National Organic Program." *The Agribusiness Examiner.*
    Issue #367, Aug 23, 2004; accessed Jan 25, 2005;
    http://www.organicconsumers.org/organic/usda.cfm

Krumm, Susan. "Refining process has sweet ending." *Lawrence
    Journal-World,* June 13, 2001; accessed Jan. 20, 2005,
    http://ljworld.com/section/cookingqa/story/55875

Langeland, Terje. "Tainted Meat, Tainted Money: Consumer
    groups decry coziness between government, agribusiness."

Colorado Springs Independent online edition, Aug. 1-7, 2002; accessed Feb. 20, 2005, http://www.csindy.com/csindy/2002-08-01/cover2.html

Langley, Gill, MA, Ph.D. *Vegan Nutrition: A Survey Of Research.* Oxford: The Vegan Society, 1988.

"The Latest In Cancer: 'White Meat' Linked to Colon Cancer." Pcrm.org, Winter 99; accessed March 28, 2005, http://www.pcrm.org/magazine/GM99Winter9.html

Leake, Jonathon. "The rich and emotional lives of cows." News.com; accessed Feb. 28, 2005, http://www.news.com/au/story/0,10117,12390397-13762,00.html

Mason, Jim and Peter Singer. *Animal Factories.* New York: Crown, 1990.

McCaleb, Rob. "Stevia Leaf—Too Good To Be Legal?" Herb Research Foundation, accessed Feb. 14, 2005, http://www.holisticmed.com/sweet/stv-faq.txt

"Men's Health Warns of Foods You Should Never Eat." Peta.org, accessed March 23, 2005, http://www.peta.org/feat/menshealth/

Mercola, Joseph, M.D. with Alison Rose Levy. *The No-Grain Diet: Conquer Carbohydrate Addiction and Stay Slim for Life.* New York: Dutton, 2003.

Mercola, Joseph, M.D. "The Potential Dangers of Sucralose." vitaminlady.com; accessed Sept. 9, 2005, http://www.vitaminlady.com/articles/sucralose.asp

Mercola, Joseph, M.D. "The Secret Dangers of Splenda (Sucralose), an Artificial Sweetener," Dec. 3, 2000; accessed Feb. 20, 2005, http://www.mercola.com/2000/dec/3/sucralose_dangers.htm

Mercola, Joseph, M.D. "Splenda—Here We Go Again." July 21, 2004; accessed Feb. 12, 2005, http://www.mercola.com/fcgi/pf/2004/jul/21/splenda.htm

Mercola, Joseph, M.D. "US 'Food Pyramid' Invalid as It was Made by Experts with Conflicts of Interest." Nov. 19, 2000; accessed Jan. 10, 2005, http://www.mercola.com/2000/nov/19/food_pyramid.htm

"Milk Sucks." Peta.org.; milksucks.com, accessed March 12, 2005, http://www.milksucks.com/

Mindell, Earl R., Ph.D. with Hester Mundis. *Earl Mindell's New Vitamin Bible.* New York, Boston: Warner, 2004.

"Molasses." Everything2com, Oct. 2, 2003; accessed Feb. 2, 2005, http://www.everything2.com/index.pl?node=molasses

"Molasses nutrition data." Nutritiondata.com, accessed March 3, 2005, http://www.nutritiondata.com/facts-001-02s04at.html

Murray, Rich. "How Aspartame Became Legal-The Timeline." Dec. 24, 2002; accessed March 5, 2005, http://www.quantumbalancing.com/news/aspartameapproved.htm

Myss, Caroline, Ph.D. *Anatomy of the Spirit: The Seven Stages of Power and Healing.* New York: Three Rivers, 1996.

"National Cattleman's Beef Association Pays for Sadistic Anti-Vegan 'Study.'" Vegsource Interactive Inc., accessed Feb. 22, 2005, http://www.vegsource.com/articles2/ncbs_vegan_study.htm

"National Soft Drink Association Protest (Summary)" Congressional Record-Senate, March 11, 2005; accessed Jan. 20, 2005, http://www.dorway.com/nsda.txt

"Nation's Largest Organic Dairy Brand, Horizon, Accused of Violating Organic Standards." The Cornucopia Institute, Feb. 16, 2005, accessed March 2, 2005, http://www.organicconsumers.org/organic/horizon21705.cfm

"Natural Sweeteners." Natural Nutrition, accessed Feb. 2, 2005, http://www.livrite.com/sweeten.htm

"Natural Sweetener-Safe for Diabetics," accessed Feb. 15, 2005, http://www.primalnature.com/stevia.html

Ness, Carol. "Organic Food: Outcry Over Rule Changes that Allow More Pesticides, Hormones." The San Francisco Chronicle, May 22, 2004, accessed March 2, 2005, http://www.common-dreams.org/cgi-bin/print.cgi?file=/headlines04/0522-09.htm

Nestle, Marion. *Food Politics: How the Food Industry Influences Nutrition and Health*. California: University of California, 2000.

Notmilk.com. March 5, 2005, http://notmilk.com/forum/526.html

"OCA and Environmental Groups Sue USDA to Enforce Strict Standards: Environmental Groups Back Harvey Lawsuit."

Organic Business News. December 2004, Vol. 16, no. 12; accessed Jan. 12, 2005, http://organicconsumers.org/organic/lawsuit010505.cfm

"Organic Industry and Consumers Celebrate USDA Reversal on Non-Food National Organic Standards" press release, May 26, 2004; accessed Feb. 10, 2005, http://www.westonaprice.org/federalupdate/aa2004/infoalert_052604.html

Pert, Candace B., Ph.D. *Molecules of Emotion.* New York: Scribner, 1997

"Pigs: Smart Animals at the Mercy of the Pork Industry." Peta.org, accessed March 3, 2005, http://www.peta.org.factsheet/files/FactsheetDisplay.asp?ID=119

Pyevich, Caroline. "Sugar and other sweeteners: Do they contain animal products?" *Vegetarian Journal.* Volume XVI, no. 2, March/April 1997; accessed Feb. 25, 2005, http://www.stanford.edu/group/vegan/sweeteners.htm

Robbins, John. *Diet For A New America.* Walpole: Stillpoint, 1987.

Roberts, H.J., M.D. "The Bressler Report." *Sun Sentinel Press;* accessed Feb. 22, 2005, http://www.presidiotex.com/bressler/

"Salts That Heal and Salts That Kill." Curezone.com, accessed March 14, 2005, http://www.curezone.com/foods/saltcure.asp

Savona, Natalie. *The Kitchen Shrink: Foods and Recipes for a Healthy Mind.* London: Duncan Baird, 2003.

Schlosser, Eric. "The Cow Jumped Over the U.S.D.A." *New York Times,* Jan. 2, 2004; accessed March 1, 2005, http://www.commondreams.org/views04/0102-06.htm

Schlosser, Eric. *Fast Food Nation: The Dark Side of the All-American Meal.* New York: Perennial, 2002.

Severson, Kim. "Sugar coated: We're drowning in high fructose corn syrup. Do the risks go beyond our waistline?" *San Francisco Chronicle* on the Web, Feb. 18, 2004; accessed Feb. 10, 2005, http://www.sfgate.com/cgi-bin/article.cgi?f=/chroni-cle/ archive/2004/02/18/FDGS24VKMH1.DTL

Simon, Michele. "Dairy Industry Propaganda: Tale of Two Mega-Campaigns." Originally published at Vegan.com, April 1999; accessed Feb. 7, 2005, http://www.informedeating.org/ docs/dairy_industry_propaganda.html

Simon, Michele. "Misery on the Menu: The National School Lunch Program." Originally published in *The Animal's Agenda,* September/October 1998; accessed Feb. 7, 2005, http://www.informedeating.org/docs/misery_on_the_menu.ht ml

Simon, Michele, JD, MPH. "The Politics of Meat and Dairy." Earthsave.org, accessed Jan. 26, 2005, http://wwwearthsave.org/news/polsmd.htm

"Soft Drinks, High-Fructose Corn Syrup Promote Diabetes, Says Study." March 10, 2005; accessed March 15, 2005, http://www.newstarget.com/002584

Squires, Sally. "Sweet but Not So Innocent?" *The Washington Post* on the Web, March 11, 2003; accessed 18 Feb 2005, http://www.washingtonpost.com/ac2/wp-dyn/A8003-2003Mar10?language=printer

Steinman, David. *Diet for a Poisoned Planet: How to Choose Safe Foods for You and Your Family.* New York: Harmony, 1990.

"Sugar Blues." Natural Nutrition, accessed Feb. 2, 2005, http://livrite.com/sugar1.htm

"Surgeon General Asks: Got Bones?" Gotmilk.com, Oct. 26, 2004; accessed March 21, 2005, http://www.gotmilk.com/news/news_035.html

"10 Reasons to Avoid Acidosis." Poly MVA Survivors.com, accessed March 28, 2005, http://polymvasurvivors.com/4corners_coral.html

"Two New Studies Sour Milk's Image." Pcrm.org, Dec. 3, 2004; accessed March 20, 2005, http://www.pcrm.org/news/release041202.html

"Unhealthy link between caffeine and diabetes." CBC Health & Science News, Jan. 9, 2002; accessed Feb. 20, 2005, http://www.cbc.ca/story/science/national/2002/01/09/caffeine_diabetes020109.html

"The U.S. Food and Drug Administration (FDA) and the glutamate industry." July 12, 2004; accessed Feb. 4, 2005, http://www.truthinlabeling.org/legislators2.html

"USDA Cover-Up of Mad Cow Cases." organicconsumers.org,
      May 10, 2005; accessed June 1, 2005,
      http://www.organicconsumers.org/bytes/051005.cfm

"USDA won't stop use of illegal hormones in the veal industry:
      cancer rates skyrocket in humans." Jan. 26, 2005; accessed
      Jan. 27, 2005, http://www.newstarget.com/z0001067.html

U.S. Department Of Agriculture. APIS Veterinary Services.
      January 2005. "National Animal Identification System:
      Goal and Visions," accessed March 12, 2005,
      http://animalid.usda.gov/ nais/about/nais_overview_fact-
      sheet.shtml

U.S. Department Of Agriculture. "About USDA"; accessed March
      12, 2005, http://www.usda.gov/wps/portal/!ut/p/_s.7_0_A/7
      _0_1OB?navtype=MA&navid=ABOUT_USDA

U.S. Department of Health and Human Services. "Symptoms
      Attributed to Aspartame in Complaints Submitted to the
      FDA." April 20, 1995; accessed Feb. 22, 2005,
      http://www.presidiotex.com/ aspar-
      tame/Facts/92_Symptoms/92_symptoms.html

Van Straten, Michael. *Super Detox.* London: Quadrille, 2003.

"Vegan FAQs." Vegan Action, accessed Jan. 20, 2005,
      "http://www.vegan.org/FAQs/

"Vegetarian and Vegan Famous Athletes." Veggie.org, accessed
      March 21, 2005,

http://veggie.org/veggie/famous.veg.athletes.shtml

Waehner, Paige. "Exercise Bulimia, the New Eating Disorder," accessed March 5, 2005, http://exercise.about.com/cs/exercisehealth/ a/exercisebulimia_p.htm

Wangen, Stephen N.D. "Food Allergy Solutions Review." FoodAllergySolutions.com, July 2003; accessed March 28, 2005, http://www.foodallergysolutions.com/food-allergy-news0307.html

Weil, Andrew, M.D. *Natural Health, Natural Medicine.* Boston: Houghton Mifflin, 1998.

Weil, Andrew, M.D. "Does Soy Have a Dark Side?" Dr. Andrew Weil's Self Healing, March 2003; accessed March 15, 2005, http://www.drweilselfhealing.com

Weiss, Suzanne E. *Reader's Digest: Foods that Harm, Foods that Heal: An A-Z Guide to Safe and Healthy Eating.* Pleasantville: The Reader's Digest Association Inc., 1997.

Whitney, Eleanor Noss, and Sharon Rady Rolfes. *Understanding Nutrition,* 8th ed. Belmont: Wadsworth, 1999.

Wijers-Hasegawa, Yumi. "Bayer's GE Crop Herbicide, Glufosinate, Causes Brain Damage." Goldenharvestorganics.com, accessed March 28, 2005, http://www.ghorganics.com/COMMON%20PESTICIDE%20CAUSES%20AGGRESSION%20&%20BRAIN%20DAMAGE.htm

Endnotes

1 Steinman, *Diet for a Poisoned Planet,* 166-7.

2 Young, *The pH Miracle: Balance Your Diet,* Reclaim Your Health, 90.

3 Gold, "Formaldehyde Poisoning from Aspartame."

4 Steinman, 190.

5 Ibid., 191.

6 "Caffeine," ecuremelife.com.

7 "Unhealthy link found between caffeine and diabetes," CBC Health & Science News.

8 Young, 51.

9 Ibid., 24-5.

10 Howell, "Why Choose Organic Coffee?"

11 Steinman, 355.

12 Young, 75.

13 Waehner, "Exercise Bulimia, the New Eating Disorder."

14 Pert, *Molecules of Emotion,* 321-22.

15 Whitney and Rolfes, *Understanding Nutrition*, 44

16 Diamond, *Fit for Life*, 65-69.

17 Chandel, "Sweet Poison," The Sunday Tribune Spectrum, tribuneindia.com.

18 "Sugar Blues," Natural Nutrition, livrite.com.

19 Chandel.

20 "Soft Drinks, High-Fructose Corn Syrup Promote Diabetes, Says Study," newstarget.com.

21 Davis, "A Tale of Two Sweeteners: Aspartame & Stevia," suewidemark.netfirms.com.

22 "Natural Sweeteners, Natural Nutrition, livrite.com.

23 Gold, "Common Toxic and Substances to Avoid," holisticmed.com.

24 Murray, "How Aspartame Became Legal—The

Timeline," quantumbalancing.com.

[25] Ibid.

[26] Ibid.

[27] "Department of Health and Human Services-Symptoms Attributed to Aspartame in Complaints Submitted to the FDA," U.S. Department of Health and Human Services, presidiotex.com.

[28] Johnson,"Aspartame . . . A Killer!" *The Sunday Express London,* newfrontier.com.

[29] Hasselberger, "Aspartame: RICO Complaint filed Against Nutra-Sweet, ADA, Monsanto," newmediaexplorer.org.

[30] Young, 89.

[31] Gold, "The Bitter Truth about Artificial Sweeteners," truthcampaign.ukf.net.

[32] *Webster's New World Dictionary* (1982), s.v. "saccharin."

[33] Mercola, "The Potential Dangers of Sucralose,

vitaminlady.com

[34] Mercola, "Splenda—Here We Go Again," mercola.com.

[35] Mercola, "The Potential Dangers of Sucralose."

[36] Burros, "Splenda's 'Sugar' Claim Unites Odd Couple of Nutrition Wars," *New York Times,* skyhen.org.

[37] Young, 50-51.

[38] Ibid., 14-15.

[39] "10 Reasons To Avoid Acidosis."

[40] Young, 51-52.

[41] Weil, *Natural Health, Natural Medicine,* 27.

[42] Fuhrman, *Eat to Live,* 98.

[43] Ibid., 95.

[44] Robbins, *Diet for a New America,* 290.

[45] Grace, *A Way Out,* 8-9.

[46] Ibid., 8-10.

[47] Steinman, 76.

[48] Brownlee, "The Beef about UTIs."

[49] Steinman, 73.

50 Cousens, *Conscious Eating,* 433.

51 Ibid., 315.

52 Ibid., 322.

53 Ibid., 313.

54 Wijers-Hasegawa, "Bayer's GE Crop Herbicide, Glufosinate, Causes Brain Damage."

55 Cousens, 438.

56 Steinman, 90.

57 Ibid., 80.

58 "Men's Health Warns of Foods You Should Never Eat," Peta.org.

59 Baillie-Hamilton, *The Body Restoration Plan,* 36.

60 Ibid., 34-5.

61 "FDA Approved Animal Drug Products," FDA 'Green Book' section.

62 Mason and Singer, *Animal Factories,* 75.

63 "The Latest In Cancer: 'White Meat' Linked to Colon Cancer," pcrm.org; Singh PN, Fraser GE. Dietary risk factors for colon cancer in a low-risk population. Am J Epidem 1998; 148:761-74.

64 Ibid.

65 Robbins, 303.

66 Steinman, 73.

67 Ibid., 313-14.

68 "Fish and Shellfish: Contamination Problems Preclude Inclusion in the Dietary Guidelines for Americans," pcrm.org, Spring 2004.

69 Weiss, *Reader's Digest: Foods that Harm, Foods that Heal,* 345.

70 Weil, *Natural Health, Natural Medicine,* 37.

71 Weil, "Does Soy Have a Dark Side?" drandrewweil-selfhealing.com.

72 Diamond, *Fit For Life II,* 242.

73 Cousens, 479.

74 "10 Reasons To Avoid Acidosis," PolyMVASurvisors.com.

75 Diamond, *Fit For Life II,* 243.

[76] "Milk Sucks," milksucks.com.

[77] Ibid.

[78] Ibid.

[79] Cohen, "The Essence of Betrayal," notmilk.com.

[80] Wangen "Food Allergy Solutions Review," FoodAllergySolutions.com.

[81] "Milk Sucks: Find Out more," milksucks.com.

[82] "Two New Studies Sour Milk's Image," pcrm.org.

[83] Robbins, 150.

[84] Steinman, 131-132.

[85] "Milk Sucks," milksucks.com.

[86] Cousens, 478.

[87] Steinman, 122.

[88] Holford, *The Optimum Nutrition Bible*, 42.

[89] Robbins, 164.

[90] Cousens, 316.

[91] Weiss, 87.

[92] Eisnitz, *Slaughterhouse,* 20, 24-25, 31.

[93] Ibid, 66.

[94] Ibid., 69-70.

[95] Ibid., 126-133.

[96] Ibid., 29.

[97] Ibid., 20, 28-29.

[98] Ibid., 71.

[99] Ibid., 166.

[100] Ibid.

[101] Ibid.

[102] Ibid.

[103] Ibid., front jacket.

[104] Ibid., 124.

[105] Ibid., 82.

[106] Ibid., 125.

[107] Ibid., 87.

[108] Ibid., 84.

[109] Ibid., 91.

[110] Ibid., 93.

[111] Ibid., 130.

[112] Ibid., 132.

[113] Ibid., 132-133.

[114] Ibid., 144-145.

[115] Ibid., 145.

[116] Ibid., 93.

[117] Ibid., 133.

[118] Ibid., 140-141.

[119] Ibid., 172.

[120] Ibid.

[121] Ibid., 173.

[122] Ibid., 174.

[123] Ibid., 175.

[124] Leake, "The rich emotional & intellectual lives of cows."

[125] "The Hidden Lives of Chickens," Peta.org.

[126] "Pigs: Smart Animals at the Mercy of the Pork Industry," Peta.org.

[127] "Fish Feel Pain," Fishinghurts.com.

[128] "Free-Range Eggs and Meat: Conning Consumers?" Peta.org.

[129] "Investigation Reveals Slaughter Horrors at Agriprocessors," Peta.org.

[130] Eisnitz, "Ask the Experts," Peta.org.

[131] Eisnitz, *Slaughterhouse,* 125.

[132] Brown, e-mail.

[133] "Animal Friendly Quotes," Peta.org.

[134] "Everything you need to eat right for your health," Peta.org.

[135] "Factory Farming: Environmental Consequences," Animalalliance.ca.

[136] Cook, "Environmental Hogwash," inthese-times.com.

[137] Cousens, 442.

[138] Young, 82-3.

[139] Howell, *Enzyme Nutrition,* 4.

[140] Ibid., 4-5.

[141] Cousens, 299.

[142] Ibid., 299.

[143] Ibid., 313.

[144] Ibid., 417.

[145] Holford, 29.

[146] Cousens, 312.

[147] Ibid.

[148] Holford, 41.

[149] Cousens, 587.

[150] "Vegetarian and Vegan Famous Athletes," Veggie.org.

151 Weil, *Natural Health, Natural Medicine,* 30.

152 Young, 68.

153 Whitney and Rolfes, *Understanding Nutrition,* 8th ed., 130-31.

154 Kamen, *New Facts About Fiber,* 43-85.

155 Ibid., 14.

156 Ibid., 10.

157 Holford, 109.

158 "About USDA," U.S. Department of Agriculture.

159 Schlosser, "The Cow Jumped Over the U.S.D.A," *New York Times,* commondreams.org.

160 Simon, "The Politics of Meat and Dairy," earthsave.org.

161 Langeland, "Tainted Meat, Tainted Money: Consumer groups decry coziness between government, agribusiness," *Colorado Springs Independent online.*

162 Schlosser, "The Cow Jumped Over the U.S.D.A."

163 Ibid.

164 Ibid.

165 "National Animal Identification System: Goal and Vision," U.S. Department of Agriculture APIS Veterinary Services.

166 Ibid.

167 "USDA Cover-Up of Mad Cow Cases," organic-consumers.org

168 "USDA won't stop use of illegal hormones in the veal industry: cancer rates skyrocket in humans," newstarget.com.

169 Nestle, *Food Politics: How the Food Industry Influences Nutrition and Health,* 73.

170 Ibid.

171 "Common Dairy Digestive Under-Recognized and Under-Diagnosed in Minorities," Johnson & Johnson.

172 Simon, "Dairy Industry Propaganda: Tale of Two Mega-Campaigns," origi-

nally published on vegan.com.

173 "Surgeon General Asks: Got Bones?" gotmilk.com.

174 Simon, "Dairy Industry Propaganda."

175 "Surgeon General Asks: Got Bones?"

176 "About USDA."

177 Simon, "The Politics of Meat and Dairy."

178 Simon, "Misery on the Menu: The National School Lunch Program," originally published in *The Animal's Agenda,* informedeating.org.

179 Schlosser, *Fast Food Nation,* 219-20.

180 Simon, "Misery on the Menu."

181 "Food and Nutrition Assistance Programs," Economic Research Service, USDA.gov.

182 Simon, "The Politics of Meat and Dairy."

183 Ness, "Organic Food: Outcry Over Rule Changes that Allow More Pesticides, Hormones," *The San Francisco Chronicle,* commondreams.org.

184 "Organic Industry and Consumers Celebrate USDA Reversal on Non-Food National Organic Standards," The Weston A. Price Foundation, weston-aprice.org.

185 Harris, "Organic Consumers Association (OCA), the Nation's Largest Organic Consumer Group Denounces Degradation of Organic Food Standards by Congress," about.com.

186 "Organic Industry and Consumers Celebrate USDA Reversal on Non-Food National Organic Standards."

187 Krebs, "USDA Accused of Allowing 'Sham' Certifiers to Participate in National organic Program," *The Agribusiness Examiner.*

188 "OCA and Environmental Groups Sue USDA to

Enforce Strict Standards: Environmental Groups Back Harvey Lawsuit," Organic Business News, organicconsumers.org.

[189] "Nation's Largest Organic Dairy Brand, Horizon, Accused of Violating Organic Standards," The Cornucopia Institute.

[190] Simon, "The Politics of Meat and Dairy."

[191] Green, "Not Milk: The USDA, Monsanto, and the U.S. Dairy Industry," *LiP Magazine.*

[192] Ibid.

[193] "The U.S. Food and Drug Administration (FDA) and the glutamate industry," truthinlabeling.org.

[194] "Food Additives," new-fitness.com.

[195] "Banned as Human Food, StarLink Corn Found in Food Aid," *Environmental News Service.*

[196] Greger, "Rocket Fuel in Milk," Dr.Greger.org.

[197] Ibid.

[198] Cook.

[199] Ibid.

[200] Schlosser, *Fast Food Nation,* 210-214.

[201] Cook.

[202] Barnard, *Breaking the Food Seduction,* 17-19.

[203] Ibid., 20-21.

[204] Ibid., 50-51.

[205] Ibid., 52.

[206] Ibid., 53.

[207] Diamond, *Fit For Life II,* 245.

[208] Barnard, 99-102.

[209] Ibid., 111-14.

[210] Cousens, 231-32.

[211] Van Straten, *Super Detox,* 12.

[212] Cousens, 231-34.

[213] Ibid., 232.

[214] Van Staten, 13.

[215] Cousens, 233.

[216] Ibid., 234.

[217] Ibid., 231.

[218] Mindell, *Earl Mindell's New*

Vitamin Bible, 39-127.

[219] Boschen, "Cycles of the Body," thejuiceguy.com.

[220] Farlow, *Food Additives: A Shopper's Guide To What's Safe & What's Not,* 7-75; "Caring Consumer Guide," Peta.org.

[221] Weil, *Natural Health, Natural Medicine,* 17-18.

[222] Holford, 24.

[223] Farlow, 41-2.

[224] "Salts that Heal and Salts that Kill," curezone.com.

[225] "National Cattlemen's Beef Association Pays for Sadistic Anti-Vegan 'Study,' " vegsource.com.

[226] Myss, *Anatomy of the Spirit,* 53-55.

P.S. Wait! We have a confession to make. We really couldn't care less about being skinny. Don't get scared or upset; you will definitely lose weight if you adopt the *Skinny Bitch* lifestyle. However, our real hope is for you to become healthy. We don't want anyone to be obsessed with getting skinny. When you eat right and exercise, you feel strong and healthy and confident. You start loving your body—not because you lose weight—but because you feel great. It's an inside job. You're finally treating your body like the temple it is.

Comparison is the thief of joy. No matter what we do, most of us will never look like supermodels or celebrities. And accepting that will make our lives a whole lot better. So what if there is only one standard of beauty perpetuated by Hollywood that you don't fit into? Don't buy into that bullshit. Take excellent care of the body you were blessed with, and love, love, love it!

—Rory Freedman and Kim Barnouin